Acting, Spectating, and the Unconscious

From Aristotle's theory of tragic *katharsis* onwards, theorists of the theatre have long engaged with the question of what spectatorship entails. This question has, directly or indirectly, often been extended to the investigation of acting.

Acting, Spectating, and the Unconscious approaches the unconscious aspects of spectatorship and acting afresh. Interweaving psychoanalytic descriptions of processes such as transference, unconscious phantasy and alpha-function with an in-depth survey of theories of spectating and acting from thinkers such as Brecht, Diderot, Rousseau and Plato, Maria Grazia Turri offers a significant insight into the emotions inherent in both the art of the actor, and the spectator's experience.

A compelling investigation of the unconscious communication between spectators and actors, this volume is a must-read for students and scholars fascinated by theatre spectatorship.

Maria Grazia Turri is an independent theatre scholar, and a psychiatrist at the University of Oxford. She completed her PhD in Drama at the University of Exeter in 2015. In her research, she applies psychoanalysis to the analysis of theatre processes.

Routledge Advances in Theatre and Performance Studies

For a full list of titles in this series, please visit www.routledge.com

39 Play, Performance, and Identity
How Institutions Structure Ludic Spaces
Edited by Matt Omasta and Drew Chappell

40 Performance and Phenomenology
Traditions and Transformations
Edited by Maaike Bleeker, Jon Foley Sherman, and Eirini Nedelkopoulou

41 Historical Affects and the Early Modern Theater
Edited by Ronda Arab, Michelle M. Dowd, and Adam Zucker

42 Food and Theatre on the World Stage
Edited by Dorothy Chansky and Ann Folino White

43 Global Insights on Theatre Censorship
Edited by Catherine O'Leary, Diego Santos Sánchez, and Michael Thompson

44 Mainstream AIDS Theatre, the Media, and Gay Civil Rights
Making the Radical Palatable
Jacob Juntunen

45 Rewriting Narratives in Egyptian Theatre
Translation, Performance, Politics
Edited by Sirkku Aaltonen and Areeg Ibrahim

46 Theatre, Exhibition, and Curation
Displayed and Performed
Georgina Guy

47 Acting, Spectating, and the Unconscious
A psychoanalytic perspective on unconscious processes of identification in the theatre
Maria Grazia Turri

Acting, Spectating, and the Unconscious

A psychoanalytic perspective on unconscious processes of identification in the theatre

Maria Grazia Turri

Routledge
Taylor & Francis Group
LONDON AND NEW YORK

First published 2017 by Routledge

2 Park Square, Milton Park, Abingdon, Oxon, OX14 4RN
605 Third Avenue, New York, NY 10017

Routledge is an imprint of the Taylor & Francis Group, an informa business

First issued in paperback 2020

British Library Cataloguing in Publication Data
A catalogue record for this book is available from the British Library

Library of Congress Cataloging in Publication Data
Names: Turri, Maria Grazia, author.
Title: Acting, spectating, and the unconscious : a psychoanalytic perspective on unconscious processes of identification in the theatre / Maria Grazia Turri.
Description: New York : Routledge, 2017. | Series: Routledge advances in theatre and performance studies
Identifiers: LCCN 2016023532 | ISBN 9781138699243 (hardback) | ISBN 9781315517339 (ebook)
Subjects: LCSH: Theater audiences—Psychology. | Acting—Psychological aspects. | Theater and society. | Subconsciousness in art.
Classification: LCC PN1590.A9 T87 2017 | DDC 792.01—dc23
LC record available at https://lccn.loc.gov/2016023532

ISBN: 978-1-138-69924-3 (hbk)
ISBN: 978-0-367-73665-1 (pbk)

Typeset in Times New Roman
by Apex CoVantage, LLC

To my family

'Che vuol dire che l'uomo ama tanto l'imitazione e l'espressione ec. delle passioni? [. . .] non è dunque la sola verità dell'imitazione, né la sola bellezza e dei soggetti, e di essa, che l'uomo desidera, ma la forza, l'energia, che lo metta in attività, e lo faccia sentire gagliardamente. L'uomo odia l'inattività, e di questa vuol esser liberato dalle arti belle'.

Giacomo Leopardi, *Zibaldone* (1822), 2361–2362

[Why does man love mimesis and the expression of the passions? [. . .] it is not then just the truth in mimesis, nor just its beauty or that of its objects, which man longs for, but that power, that energy, that sets him in action, and makes him feel with vigour. Man hates inactivity, and from it he wishes to be freed by art.]

Contents

A note on the text

All quotations are given in English in the main text; the original is provided in an endnote when the specific wording is relevant to my discussion. For quotations from works for which an English version is not available, the translation into English is mine; in such cases, the original is always given in an endnote.

I have used the official style required for citations from 'The Standard Edition of the Complete Psychological Works of Sigmund Freud'; this entails that each work is quoted separately. I have followed a similar convention for what concerns Klein's and Brecht's writings, listing each essay as single entries. Although I have used the collected versions of their works, these writings were originally published individually. I believe that my choice will enable readers to refer immediately to the source text and thus help them to follow my argument with greater precision.

I have given some consideration to the question of how to use gender pronouns when writing in general terms, so as to avoid using the masculine as the universal gender. Any convention has got its limitations; my choice has been partly practical in terms of helping the reader to navigate the text more easily. I have used the feminine for the actor and for the analyst, and the masculine for the spectator and for the patient, and this convention mirrors the use of the feminine for the mother and the masculine for the baby, when I am talking about the mother-baby relationship. Quotations or specific examples necessarily, and happily, escape from this system.

Acknowledgements

I wish to thank Professor David Wiles, for having given me the opportunity to conduct this research as a PhD student at the Department of Theatre and Drama at Royal Holloway and at the Drama Department at the University of Exeter, and for his advice and encouragement. I am grateful to my family for having lent me more than a hand during the writing of the book. This research would not have been possible without access to the extraordinary resources of the Bodleian and Taylor Institution Libraries in Oxford, which have been for so many years like a second home.

Chapter 1

Theorizing theatre spectatorship

Starting with Brecht

Theatre masters and theorists of the distant or less distant past have always concerned themselves with spectators. Their preoccupations have been multiple: it might have been to dictate a measure for playwriting or a measure for acting, or it might have been to justify their condemnation of theatre or to defend their reformation of it. While the twentieth century has been particularly fertile in its attempts to theoretically redefine and practically reconfigure the relationship between theatre and audience, the audience has persistently been the point of reference against which theatre has defined itself (Freshwater, 2009). Brecht is exemplary in founding his criticism of conventional theatre and his reform in the direction of the epic theatre on his preoccupation with the effects of theatre on spectators.

Brecht maintains that the audience's experience in conventional theatre amounts to *katharsis* and he employs the epithet of 'Aristotelian theatre' to illustrate theatre's ability to entice the audience into an identification with the characters of the play through which spectators are transported into the characters' emotional states. Although the word 'identification' does not feature in Aristotle's text, Brecht decidedly interprets *katharsis* as entailing emotional identification. To define emotional identification, he uses the German word '*Einfühlung*', which literally means 'feeling into', and whose most common English translation is 'empathy'. Brecht (1951: 184) disapproves of emotional identification, or the 'empathy operation', as he will call it, on the basis that it leads the audience to a passive and uncritical submission to the situation presented by the play. In fact, by maintaining that the audience's emotional identification amounts to becoming a passive sufferer of the art work (Brecht, 1930), he establishes an abiding correlation between the concepts of emotional identification and passivity. Such notion will remain engrained in contemporary theories of spectatorship.

An exemplary post-Brechtian description of theatrical empathy is given by Augusto Boal (2008: 30–31) in his *Theatre of the Oppressed*, where following Brecht's lesson, he equates emotional identification with passive surrendering to the feelings and behaviours of the character:

> From the moment the performance begins, a relationship is established between the character, especially the protagonist, and the spectator. This relationship

> has well defined characteristics: the spectator assumes a passive attitude and delegates the power of action to the character. Since the character resembles us (as Aristotle indicates), we live *vicariously* all his stage experiences. Without acting, we feel that we are acting. We love and hate when the character loves and hates.

The relationship between empathy and passivity is grounded in Brecht's interpretation of *katharsis*. In line with the prevailing rendition of his times, he translates *katharsis* with '*Reinigung*', the German word for 'purgation'. While typically such purgation was intended to apply to the spectator's emotions, Brecht's distinctive reading extends it to mean that the spectator will undergo, through empathy, a wider cleansing not limited to his emotions, but comprising any tendency to political or social activism, or even awareness of their possibility. Because according to Brecht (1963: 151) no theatre can ever be un-political, the apparently innocuous 'purpose of pleasure' (Brecht, 1949: 181) at the heart of Aristotelian theatre is a powerful device for social oppression. Society uses this kind of entertainment 'to reproduce itself' (Brecht, 1930: 34) by keeping the audience in a state of emotional intoxication which numbs their consciousness or dissent. In his extension of the Brechtian interpretation of *katharsis*, Boal (2008: 29) defines it as 'the purification of the extraneous, undesirable element which prevents the character from achieving his ends. This extraneous element is contrary to the law; it is a social fault, a political deficiency'. Therefore, *katharsis* is the instrument through which Aristotelian theatre becomes an 'extremely powerful poetic-political system for intimidation of the spectator, for elimination of the "bad" or illegal tendencies of the audience' (Boal, 2008: 3).

Brecht's perception of *katharsis* as a means to political subjugation implies a profound mistrust for the value of the spectator's emotional identification with the characters of the play, evocative of Rousseau's. In his *Lettre à d'Alembert*, the French philosopher offers a gripping and authoritative precursor to Brecht's conception of *katharsis*, when he asks what the Aristotelian pity amounts to:

> Some will say that tragedy excites the audience to pity by means of terror: be it so; but what sort of pity is this? [. . .] a barren pity, fed with a few tears, and never productive of the least act of humanity. Thus did the bloody Sylla weep at misfortunes, of which he himself was not the cause. Thus did the tyrant of Pherae hide himself at the play, lest he should be seen to sigh with Andromache and Priamus, while he felt not the least concern at the cries of so many unfortunates, who were every day butchered by his orders.
>
> (Rousseau, 1759: 24)

Emotional identification with the characters of the play functions as an insulated experience which at the worst is corrupting, at the best is immaterial to human morality. In this sense Susan Bennett (1997: 1), in her theory of spectatorship as cultural phenomenon, can speak of the 'productive and emancipated spectator', as a spectator 'who can think and act', as opposed to a passive spectator who feels. The invention of the epic theatre is precisely Brecht's attempt at transforming spectatorship from what he considered a passive emotional process founded on empathy to an active intellectual engagement grounded in reason and ultimately conducive to political action.

The epic theatre

Brecht developed the idea of the 'epic theatre' in the early 1920s, in the context of his activity as playwright. The concept, which 'already enjoyed some currency' in the Berlin theatre scene before Brecht appropriated it (Parker, 2014: 229) was originally dramaturgical, but Brecht soon made it pertinent to questions of acting and spectating. If Aristotelian theatre implies a correspondence between the spectator's empathy and *katharsis* intended as passivity and conformism, in order to oppose the harmful cathartic effects of theatre it is necessary to dispel the audience's empathic response. The epic theatre

> makes nothing like such a free use as does the aristotelian of the passive empathy of the spectator; it also relates differently to certain psychological effects, such as catharsis. [. . .] Anxious to teach the spectator a quite definite practical attitude, directed towards changing the world, it must begin by making him adopt in the theatre a quite different attitude from what he is used to.
>
> (Brecht, 1933: 57)

The epic theatre is characterized precisely by its ability to break the emotional identification of the spectator with the characters, through a process of alienation which will activate the audience's active and socially critical response (Brecht, 1957a: 110). For the purpose of alienation, the whole apparatus which promotes illusion is deconstructed. Titles are used to break the continuity of the play (Brecht, 1931: 43); actors' positions are organized so to avoid naturalistic grouping and to reveal instead the socio-historical context (Brecht, 1933: 58). While these and other alienation devices are controlled by the playwright or the director, it is to the actor herself and her technique that the main responsibility for the alienation effect falls.

The implicit recognition of the actor as the principal vehicle of the spectator's emotional identification with the character justifies Brecht's appeal to her to mediate a different kind of experience for the spectator. From this concern originates the idea of the *Verfremdungseffekt* or *V-effekt* (translated into English as alienation):

> It is well known that contact between audience and stage is normally made on the basis of *empathy*. [. . .] the technique producing a V-effect is the exact opposite of that aiming at empathy. The actors applying it are bound not to try to bring about the empathy operation.
>
> (Brecht, 1951: 184)[1]

In an essay dedicated to his new technique of acting, Brecht (1951) explains that the breaking of the fourth wall and the distancing of the actor from the character through 'observation', as opposed to empathy, are the synergic forces which create the *Verfremdungseffekt*. The actor portrays her character through symbolic gestures which allow her to maintain the function of actor as observer, rather than converting herself into the character through a process of emotional identification. Moreover, the function of actor as observer is fostered by her awareness of the presence of an audience who watches her. If emotional empathy is that situation in Aristotelian theatre which relies on emotional identification between actor, character and spectator, observation is the new psychological process which links actor, character and spectator in the epic theatre. As von Held (2011: 43) has argued, Brecht's definition of acting remains grounded in 'a mirroring relation between actor and spectator. If the actor emotes, so does the spectator. If the actor remains rationally self-detached, the spectator, too, will be rationally detached'. Admittedly, the V-effect still engenders a form of identification between spectator and actor, but this differs from the empathy aroused by conventional theatre at least in two ways: firstly, it is based on observation and critical detachment, and hence divested of the emotional charge of empathy; secondly, it is an identification which links actor and spectator with the exclusion of the character. The spectator is permitted to mirror the actor as she observes, and indeed the actor is permitted to invite the spectator to enter into her attitude, if not her feelings, as long as the character remains excluded from their psychological and aesthetic complicity.

It is of note that *Verfremdungseffekt* is Brecht's neologism, which he introduces in 1936, at a time when he sharpens his attention towards the function of the actor. Until then, Brecht had employed the conventional word *Entfremdung* referring to the usage of the concept in Hegel and Marx; as has been suggested, *Verfremdung* 'draws a clearer distinction between a sociological category of alienation and an aesthetic of estrangement' (von Held, 2011: 25). Whereas Marxist *Entfremdung* entails the workers' dispossession of the fruits of their labour, resulting in their estrangement from their own humanity, through Brecht's *Verfremdung* the workers can enhance their social awareness by exploiting their emotional estrangement from the characters on stage. It is by refraining from portraying the characters in an empathic way, and thus at some level depriving them of their humanity, that actors promote political consciousness. It is not surprising then that the best metaphor for the job of the actor is the eyewitness at a street accident (Brecht, 1950). The eyewitness invites bystanders to form an opinion about the accident: whilst he takes upon himself the task to demonstrate to them how the accident took place, so that they can judge of it as if they had been witnessing it with their very eyes, he has no intention or desire to press them into re-experiencing the victim's feelings as the protagonists of the tragic scene. Brecht here establishes an opposition between the victim's subjugation to feeling and the witness's propensity for judgement which features as a significant motif in contentions about acting and spectating, as we shall see particularly with reference to Diderot.

Spectatorship, emotions and the unconscious

Brecht's dichotomy between a passive and an active spectator finds some correspondence with his view of a divergence between emotional and rational engagement, grounded 'within an Enlightenment tradition of dramaturgical discourse that similarly theorizes the psychological processes at work in theatre production and perception as suspended between two poles: reason and feeling' (von Held, 2011: 38). Brecht (1957a) condemns the emotional identification of spectators with characters as a passive experience and demands that theatre find devices to break it, and thus engage the spectator's reason in active criticism of society. Deprived of the possibility for emotional identification, the audience is left to grapple with the play through their rational faculties. Accordingly, Brecht (1926: 14) specifically maintains that epic theatre appeals 'to reason'.

Brecht's (1926: 15) formulations emphasize his tendency to vilify feelings and commend reason: 'Feelings are private and limited. Against that the reason is fairly comprehensive and to be relied on'. However, as he himself explained in an interview of 1952, he never intended to ground epic theatre on the absolute opposition between emotion and reason. The epic theatre

> by no means renounces emotion, least of all the sense of justice, the urge to freedom, and righteous anger; it is so far from renouncing these that it does not even assume their presence, but tries to arouse or reinforce them. The 'attitude of criticism' which it tries to awaken in its audience cannot be passionate enough for it.
>
> (Brecht, 1952: 227)

As has been pointed out (Bennett, 1997: 29), Brecht's theatre reform does not exclude the spectator's emotional involvement; rather, the *Verfremdungseffekt* 'intervenes, not in the form of *absence* of emotion, but in the form of emotions that need not correspond to those of the character portrayed' (Brecht, 1957c: 154). In fact, the apparent ambiguity towards emotions finds a resolution if it is clarified that the undesirable emotions are those that the spectator feels in identification with the character, while the permitted or even desirable ones, are those that belong to the spectator as a detached observer of the character. Brecht (1957a: 112) distinctly illustrates this point in his essay *Theatre for Pleasure or Theatre for Instruction*, where the feelings of the spectator in the Aristotelian theatre are contrasted to those of the spectator in the epic theatre. In the first situation the spectator resonates predictably with the characters' emotions in identification with them ('I weep when they weep, I laugh when they laugh'), whereas in the epic theatre the spectator's critical detachment leads him to unforeseen insights into the characters' conditions which can in turn generate unexpected emotional reactions, even opposite ones to those of the characters ('I laugh when they weep, I weep when they laugh'). The dichotomy between passive and active spectator is therefore not precisely the opposition between emotion and reason, but rather between an emotion which arises as a reflex to an identification unmediated by reason, such as *katharsis* seems to imply, and an emotion which arises as a consequence of a deliberate critical judgement, as is the case in the epic theatre. These second kind of emotions are valuable outcomes of spectatorship, whilst those which arise from emotional identification with the characters must be impeded. This distinction ultimately entails a criticism and disavowal of unconscious emotional processes as active and useful constituents of spectatorship: psychic change and, most importantly for Brecht, the social and political awareness that ensues, is entrusted solely to the operations of reason and consciousness. In other words, Brecht's preoccupation with the opposition between feelings and reason fundamentally reflects a preoccupation with the contrast between conscious and unconscious psychic processes. As he specifies in his essay *On the Use of Music in the Epic Theatre*: 'It is a frequently recurring mistake to suppose that this – epic – kind of production simply does without all emotional effects: actually, emotions are only clarified in it, steering clear of subconscious origins and intoxicating no one' (Brecht, 1957b: 128).

Brecht was not ignorant of the existence of powerful unconscious emotions which keep the human mind under their sway; on this supposition, after all, was based his whole critique of the Aristotelian theatre. But he chose to emphasize the power of reason, sometimes simplistically overstating the aptness of reason to override emotions. Thus he constructed a model of theatre spectatorship which, in acknowledging its unconscious aspects, at one and the same time dismisses them as an object worth enquiry. Brecht's theory seemed to create, the opportunity for doing away with the very notion of *katharsis* or at least to expedite the arrival of new, '*katharsis*-free', conceptualizations of spectatorship. In particular, its emphasis on the socio-political context of theatre reception instigated a view of the audience's engagement as culturally and socially determined and prompted the surge in investigations of specific audiences, historically, culturally or socially situated. It has been argued that: 'Brecht's appropriation of the *Poetics*, which overall had little in common with Aristotle's dramatic principles, serves to attack an essential mechanism activated by the bourgeois theatre that seeks to gratify a need for catharsis' (von Held, 2011: 23). Too hastily perhaps, unconscious emotional engagement has been construed to correspond with middle-class pursuits. Focusing on the social and cultural markers of theatre reception, while in itself a groundbreaking and necessary endeavour, has also obscured questions about the common psychological elements that transcend social class and cultural variation. Ultimately, Brecht's emphasis on the socio-political aspects of reception has justified not only a condemnation but also an outright denial of unconscious aspects of spectatorship. It is therefore the principal aim of this book to enrich the discourse on theatre spectatorship with a conceptual framework grounded in psychoanalysis, in order to provide a theory and a language to describe those universal aspects of theatre reception which, embedded within our unconscious psyche, have so far been neglected.

Spectatorship and psychoanalysis

The significance of the unconscious to psychic life

Freud's greatest contribution to the study of the mind was the re-discovery of the unconscious. Not so much its discovery, but its appropriation from the realm of poetry and philosophy into the sphere of the medical sciences (Gay, 2006: 127–128). Johann Friedrich Herbart, a prominent German psychologist and philosopher, had, in the early nineteenth century, recognized the important part played by the unconscious in mental life, and Freud had been exposed to his views. Despite these antecedents, however, no one before Freud had ever examined the unconscious in detail, showing 'how it worked, how it differed from other parts of the mind, and what were its reciprocal relations with them' (Freud, 1915: 164). Freud first glanced at the unconscious through hypnosis, the technique that he had learnt from famous contemporary neurologists, such as Charcot and Bernheim (Gay, 2006: 48–51) and which, as a young doctor, he had employed in the cure of hysterical patients. Hypnosis had given him the proof that there were hidden aspects of the psyche which could be brought into focus through certain techniques:

> The 'unconscious' had, it is true, long been under discussion among philosophers as a theoretical concept; but now for the first time, in the phenomena of hypnotism, it became something actual, tangible and subject to experiment. [. . .] From a theoretical as well as from a therapeutic point of view, psychoanalysis has at its command a legacy which it has inherited from hypnotism.
>
> (Freud, 1924: 192)

Although he was left eager to understand the unconscious and its relationship to thinking and behaviour, he soon abandoned hypnosis as a technique; instead he gave birth to psychoanalysis, as a new 'science of unconscious mental processes' (Freud, 1925: 70).

During his entire career Freud remained acutely aware that his discoveries about the unconscious were running contrary to prevailing views of the mind in medical and scientific institutions of his time. As he wrote in 1926:

> Psychology had barred its own access to the region of the id by insisting on a postulate which is plausible enough but untenable: namely, that all mental acts are conscious to us – that being conscious is the criterion of what is mental, and that, if there are processes in our brain which are not conscious, they do not deserve to be called mental acts and are no concern of psychology.
>
> (Freud, 1926: 196–197)

Against the prevailing tide in medicine and psychology, he continued to examine and explain the prominence of unconscious processes within the psyche and he compared the significance of his discovery to that of Darwin's theory of evolution and of Copernicus's heliocentrism: these theories had dealt a biological and a cosmological blow to mankind's narcissism; psychoanalysis would deal them a psychological one (Freud, 1924: 221). Freud was convinced that much opposition to psychoanalysis, which is still prevailing today, sprang from resistance against the idea that an unruly unconscious holds sway over a relatively constrained conscious ego. In his criticism of what he calls Aristotelian theatre, Brecht is precisely concerned about the powerful dominance of unconscious aspects of spectatorship over conscious ones. Indeed, Brecht talks of the hypnotic state of the audience, when he describes the spectators' passive submission to the cathartic effect of a play. As I have discussed, hypnotic in Brecht's terms could be substituted for by 'unconscious'. For Brecht, the hypnotic state represents a threat to humans' rational faculties and therefore must be eluded at all costs. For Freud, the unconscious is a fundamental aspect of how human beings operate, and must therefore be turned into a new field of scientific enquiry.

The significant divergence between Freud's and Brecht's attitude towards the unconscious is illustrated by a curious instance, which can almost be construed as an indirect exchange of opinions between the two men. In his essay *The Modern Theatre is the Epic Theatre* Brecht (1930) uses a quotation from Freud, the only mention of Freud to be found among his writings on the theatre. The quote is from one of Freud's works of maturity, *Civilization and Its Discontents*, and Brecht uses it to support his claim that conventional theatre is functional to a society which employs art as a narcotic drug against critical engagement, ultimately leading to the abdication of social responsibility. The passage, following Brecht's own omissions, runs as follows:

> Life, as we find it, is too hard for us; it brings us too many pains, disappointments and impossible tasks. In order to bear it we cannot dispense with palliative measures. [. . .] There are perhaps three such measures: powerful deflections, which cause us to make light of our misery; substitutive satisfactions, which diminish it; and intoxicating substances, which make us insensitive to it. Something of the kind is indispensable. [. . .] The substitutive satisfactions, as offered by art, are illusions in contrast with reality, but they are none the less psychically effective, thanks to the role which phantasy has assumed in mental life.
>
> (Freud, 1930: 75)[2]

Freud seems to claim that art's ultimate aim is to furnish man with an escapist route into a fantasy world, and that is why, adds Brecht, art as traditionally intended, and theatre in particular, need to be radically reformed. It could be argued, in fact, that Freud's theorizing about artistic production and reception, taken at face value, corroborates Brecht's preoccupations about the function of art.

Freud had attempted his own formulation of a theory of spectatorship in an essay entitled *Psychopathic Characters on the Stage*, which he wrote in 1905 but, significantly, never published during his lifetime. Predictably departing from Aristotle's theory of tragic *katharsis*, and following the accepted nineteenth-century translation of *katharsis* as purgation, he maintained that the spectator derived pleasure from the theatre by identifying with the sufferings of the tragic hero, but with the consolation that 'firstly, it is someone other than himself who is acting and suffering on the stage, and, secondly, that after all it is only a game, which can threaten no damage to his personal security' (Freud, 1906: 306). It is striking how close this explanation is to Brecht's account of the harmful effects of the Aristotelian theatre: here Freud seems to describe precisely a passive spectator who delegates all power of action to the characters and who gains from the experience a surreptitious pleasure, in participating in sufferings which will never genuinely touch him or interest him outside the auditorium. But despite the proximity of their conclusions on spectatorship, Freud and Brecht depart from very different premises. In particular, Freud could never endorse Brecht's proposition that the unconscious can simply be bypassed through reason and conscious purpose. As he maintains: 'psychoanalysis cannot situate the essence of the psychical in consciousness, but is obliged to regard consciousness as a quality of the psychical, which may be present in addition to other qualities or may be absent' (Freud, 1923: 13). Because psychoanalysis puts the unconscious at the basis of all mental activity, including higher functions such as rational thinking, there can be no coherent picture of the operating of the mind without some description of unconscious processes.

It is of note that in *Civilization and Its Discontents*, the essay quoted by Brecht, Freud engages in a specific critique of communist ideology – possibly the reason why Brecht particularly took an interest in this work. Freud's main concern is that the communist ideology is based on the false psychological presumption that inequality and injustice among mankind is solely dependent on external or material factors. As he acknowledges:

> I have no concern with any economic criticisms of the communist system; I cannot enquire into whether the abolition of private property is expedient or advantageous. But I am able to recognize that the psychological premises on which the system is based are an untenable illusion.
>
> (Freud, 1930: 113)

Freud believes that the communist ideology fails to consider the prominence of unconscious psychic processes in determining human behaviour, and any system that ignores the unconscious foundations of social and cultural activities is flawed. Whilst Freud's theoretical view of the function of art remained somewhat narrow, seemingly justifying a negative judgement about any unconscious aesthetic engagement, his broad discoveries about the unconscious, and their extension by his disciples, provide a crucial paradigm for the enhancement of our understanding of theatre spectatorship.

Psychoanalysis in context

It has been argued (Anderson, 1980) that Freud's ideas about the unconscious are a plagiarism of those of Nietzsche's and that he built his defence of psychoanalysis as a science by denying his debt towards the intuitions of artists and philosophers. Freud, however, was well aware of the insights that literature and philosophy had contributed to the understanding of psychic functioning ahead of science in general and of psychoanalysis in particular. He writes about the merits of the creative writer: 'The description of the human mind is indeed the domain which is most his own; he has from time immemorial been the precursor of science, and so too of scientific psychology' (Freud, 1907: 43–44). Of his particular relationship to Nietzsche's philosophy, he confesses in a private letter:[3] 'I have rejected the study of Nietzsche although – no, because – it was plain that I would find insights in him very similar to psychoanalytic ones' (in Gay, 2006: 46). While the existence of the unconscious and certain aspects of its functioning had been already anticipated by artists and philosophers, Freud must be credited with creating a method of observation of unconscious processes that enabled their systematic study. The invention of psychoanalysis opened a new field of knowledge whereby the unconscious was methodically investigated through the collection of clinical data as well as methodical self-observation. It is only because of Freud's endeavours and discoveries that insights into the unconscious were accepted, although with much struggle, to bear on medicine and the treatment of mental illness. While Freud was keen for the scientific community to embrace psychoanalysis, it is well known that he was often ostracized or ridiculed by the medical and scientific establishment of his age. Incidentally, it was an age when being a Jew was not a recommendation. This contextualization may help understand why Freud may, at times, have yielded to the temptation of producing overbearing statements about psychoanalysis as a scientific discipline.

In this book, I will draw upon psychoanalytic theories which explore the unconscious mechanisms of identification at the basis of emotional development and ego-formation and I will focus mainly on the conceptualizations of Freud, Klein and Bion. Psychoanalytic descriptions of the relationship between identification and identity have been harshly judged by humanities scholars, especially from a feminist perspective. These critiques have particularly focused on Freud's formulation of the Oedipus complex, and on its further elaborations by Lacan. Butler (1999: 56), for instance, has argued that through the Lacanian perspective, the male gender comes to represent the conscious subject, while the female gender is reduced to serve the function of objectifying males' desire, thus providing a 'dialectical confirmation of its identity'. This rigid gender stereotyping resonates with some of Freud's own opinions about gender development. For instance, Freud's association of the male gender with activity and of the female one with passivity presupposes a gender-biased approach to psychology which justifies 'dividing up functions and sexual roles' (Irigaray, 1993: 36) and the unequal distribution of privileges that this entails. Although Freud's Oedipus complex gets somewhat distorted by the intense scrutiny under which it has rightly been brought, its perspective on gender identity is inherently unbalanced. Yet, many other psychoanalytic formulations of ego-development and unconscious functioning are gender-neutral. Freud's theory of transference, which I will consider in detail in Chapter 2, Klein's concept of unconscious phantasy, and Bion's theory of alpha-function, both of which I will discuss in Chapter 5, are all instances of gender-neutral psychic processes.

In my discussion of psychoanalytic theories, while departing from Freud, I will also focus on Klein's elaboration of his ideas. Although outside the remit of my discussion, it must be emphasized that Klein's development of the theory of the Oedipus complex, very much in opposition to Lacan's, vindicated the significance of the female gender, emphasizing the role of the vagina and its creative potential. Klein's insights into the operations of the unconscious are generally dissimilar to those of Lacan. Both give consideration to the development of the self in relation to the encounter with the other, a field of enquiry that Phelan (1993) rightly puts at the centre of any investigation of identification and identity; however, their perspective is very different. For Klein there is no primary self outside the encounter with the other. In this sense any primary experience is fragmented and self-less, and only through the sympathetic engagement of the other can the subject painstakingly construct his sense of self. Compared to a Lacanian perspective, whereby the female other may be construed as being exploited by the observing male subject to reinforce his self-identity, in Kleinian terms the dynamic of power is reversed: an a-gendered infant psyche is at the mercy of the maternal function. Although both male and female mature minds may perform the maternal function, the linguistic metaphor assigns to the female gender the active role of promoting the infant's psychic development. She is active; he (if we want, for the sake of simplicity, to give the baby a gender) is the passive one, at the mercy of his unconscious. The mother then is, yes, putting herself at the service of her a-gendered and vulnerable baby, but not reverentially, not in order to allow him (or her) the re-affirmation of an already established sense of self, but rather as an act of generosity that will promote the development and integration of the primitive and fragmented baby's mind. My choice of assigning the actor a female pronoun and the spectator a masculine one, is an allusion to the theory of alpha-function, which I will discuss in Chapter 5. Far from hinting at a predatory male spectator who exploits the female actor to satisfy his desire and cement his sense of self, my linguistic use of pronouns indicates a vulnerable spectator who depends on the actor's maternal function for his psychic development.

A psychoanalytic perspective of theatre spectatorship

The complexity of the theatrical performance as a system of communication which utilizes multiple sensory channels, compounded by its ephemeral status which effaces its availability for subsequent scientific enquiry, has represented one of the biggest challenges to the formulation of satisfactory theories of theatre reception and has undoubtedly contributed, historically, to the more convenient conflation of theatre with its literary texts (Elam, 1980: 4). The Prague School of semiotics overcame the assimilation of theatre within literary studies and emphasized the complexity of theatre as a system of signs, as compared to other arts, including literature, music or sculpture (Veltruský, 1981). Theatre was regarded as a global system of signification, rather than a sum of semiotic subsystems, which pointed to its unique and peculiar nature: a pluricodified and multileveled organization of heterogeneous components that are interdependent (Amossy, 1981). Although this conferred on theatre a differentiated status, the difficulty with making it the object of scientific enquiry remained.

Contemporary theatre studies have examined spectatorship from a variety of different perspectives, each focusing on a particular subsystem of signification: for instance, its socio-cultural determinants (Bennett, 1997), cognitive processes (McConachie, 2008) and embodied perceptions (Fischer-Lichte, 2008). There has instead been little attention paid to unconscious emotional aspects; this may seem surprising, given that since Aristotle and for many centuries, reflections on spectatorship generally took it for granted that the audience's emotional involvement was intrinsic to theatre reception. Considered from a psychoanalytic perspective, though, this is not unexpected because much emotional engagement happens at an unconscious level, while emotional awareness consists of the sparse epiphanies emerging from the underlying continuous flow of the unconscious. It is true that psychoanalysis has extensively been applied to the study of theatre, but this pertains nearly exclusively to the analysis of dramatic content, rather than theatrical process. Psychoanalysts as well as literary scholars have employed psychoanalytic concepts to bear on the interpretation of characters and plot: the examination of classical tragedies through the theory of the Oedipus complex by the French psychoanalyst André Green (1979) or the extensive application of various psychoanalytic constructs to the analysis of Shakespeare's plays (Brown, 2015) are only two examples of many. It was in fact Freud himself who started this line of enquiry, in drawing upon classical plays like *Oedipus Rex* for illustrating and naming the mechanisms of the unconscious mind (Freud, 1900: 261–263), and then turning his insights back to bear on the analysis of literary and dramatic texts, such as his groundbreaking interpretation of Hamlet's hesitations as an expression of the character's unresolved oedipal conflicts (Freud, 1900: 264–266). On the other hand, the application of psychoanalysis to the study of theatrical processes is uncommon (rare examples are: Nuetzel, 1999; Campbell and Kear, 2001), and it has not been drawn upon systematically to enhance our understanding of spectatorship.

My application of psychoanalysis to discover and describe unconscious aspects of spectating and acting embedded in emblematic theories of the theatre aims at enriching theatre studies with a framework and language that will complement existent approaches. Brecht's emphasis on the role of the actor in mediating the spectator's response, both at an intellectual and emotional level, rightly demands that unconscious emotional processes in both actors and spectators be examined in parallel. That is why in the course of the book I will probe the psychoanalytic perspective against theories that have considered the spectator's or the actor's emotional engagement in depth. My choice of theories has been determined first by their prominence as discourses on the relevance of emotional processes for spectating and acting, and secondly by their trans-temporal connection with Brecht. Unsurprisingly, Aristotle's theory of tragic *katharsis* represents both a pivotal point of reference for reflections on spectators' emotional engagement with theatre, and the key conception of spectatorship against which Brecht launches his invective. For what concerns theories of acting, although the twentieth century is not lacking in a rich debate and a flurry of experiments on the art of the actor, I chose to focus on Diderot's *Paradoxe sur le Comédien* and on its eighteenth-century background references, because they give thorough consideration to the significance and the modalities of the actor's emotional involvement. The *Paradoxe sur le Comédien,* with its sources, represents a point of reference for future theorists, including twentieth-century theatre masters such as Stanislavski and Copeau, and it establishes the prototype for Brecht's formulation of the epic actor.

Following this framework, in Chapter 2 I will engage with Aristotle's theory of tragic *katharsis* as the classical theory of spectatorship. I will first re-consider the theory in the context of a re-evaluation of the meaning of *mimēsis*, fear and pity. I will then describe the evolution of Freud's theory of transference from his earlier conceptualization of the 'cathartic method', the precursor to psychoanalysis. Through a comparative analysis between transference and *katharsis*, I will suggest how tragic *katharsis* may reveal the transference dynamic embedded in spectating. In Chapters 3 and 4 I will shift my attention to the actor. I will depart from Diderot's *Paradoxe* as the emblematic theory of the actor which bridges the rich eighteenth-century debate on the art of the actor to twentieth-century formulations, most notably Brecht's *Verfremdungseffekt*. In Chapter 3, I will give considerable attention to the *Paradoxe*'s contentions about the art of the actor, and I will highlight its inherent contradictions. In Chapter 4, I will turn to those eighteenth-century theoretical works on acting that constitute the background references of the *Paradoxe*. In both chapters my main focus will be the different interpretations that theorists have given of the relationship between sensibility and understanding in the art of the actor. In Chapter 5, I will illustrate the mechanisms of unconscious emotional processing from a psychoanalytic perspective, drawing upon the interrelated theories of Freud, Klein and Bion. The chapter will culminate with the description of alpha-function, the transpersonal process through which raw unconscious emotional dynamics are transformed into conscious emotional insights. In Chapter 6, I will conclude by proposing a psychoanalytic understanding of unconscious processes of spectating and acting as alpha-function. I will also explain how unconscious processes of spectatorship in alpha-function can enhance our understanding of some of the most arduous questions about theatre, such as the role of feeling in the actor's interpretation, the nature of the feedback loop between audience and actors, and the peculiar character of theatre as opposed to other arts.

Notes

1 'Der Kontakt zwischen Publikum und Bühne kommt für gewöhnlich bekanntlich auf der Basis der *Einfühlung* zustande. [. . .] Schon unsere einleitenden Bemerkungen zeigen, daß die Technik, die den V-Effekt hervorbringt, der Technik, die die Einfühlung bezweckt, diametral entgengegesetzt ist. Der Schauspieler ist durch sie gehalten, die Herbeiführung des Einfühlungsaktes nicht zu betreiben' (B. Brecht, *Schriften zum Theater. Vol. 1–4* [Frankfurt am Main: Suhrkamp Verlag, 1963], Vol. 3, pp. 156–157).

2 This English translation of Freud's words as quoted by Brecht is taken from the 'Standard Edition of the Complete Psychological Works of Sigmund Freud', as per reference, and it is therefore slightly different from Willet's own translation.

3 Freud to Lothar Bickel, June 28, 19.

Bibliography

Amossy, R. (1981) 'Semiotics and Theater: By Way of Introduction', *Poetics Today*, vol. 2, no. 3, pp. 5–10.

Anderson, L. (1980) 'Freud, Nietzsche', *Salmagundi*, vol. 47/48, pp. 3–29.

Bennett, S. (1997) *Theatre and Audiences*, London: Routledge.

Boal, A. (2008) *Theatre of the Oppressed*, translated by C.A. Leal McBride, M.-O. Leal McBride and E. Fryer, London: Pluto Press.

Brecht, B. (1926) 'Conversation with Bert Brecht', in *Brecht on Theatre: The Development of an Aesthetic*, edited and translated by J. Willett (2001), London: Methuen, pp. 14–17.

Brecht, B. (1930) 'The Modern Theatre Is the Epic Theatre', in *Brecht on Theatre: The Development of an Aesthetic*, edited and translated by J. Willett (2001), London: Methuen, pp. 33–42.

Brecht, B. (1931) 'The Literarization of the Theatre', in *Brecht on Theatre: The Development of an Aesthetic*, edited and translated by J. Willett (2001), London: Methuen, pp. 43–47.

Brecht, B. (1933) 'Indirect Impact of the Epic Theatre', in *Brecht on Theatre: The Development of an Aesthetic*, edited and translated by J. Willett (2001), London: Methuen, pp. 57–62.

Brecht, B. (1949) 'A Short Organum for the Theatre', in *Brecht on Theatre: The Development of an Aesthetic*, edited and translated by J. Willett (2001), London: Methuen, pp. 179–205.

Brecht, B. (1950) 'The Street Scene: A Basic Model for an Epic Theatre', in *Brecht on Theatre: The Development of an Aesthetic*, edited and translated by J. Willett (2001), London: Methuen, pp. 121–128.

Brecht, B. (1951) 'Short Description of a New Technique of Acting That Produces a *Verfremdung* Effect', in *Brecht on Theatre*, edited by M. Silberman, S. Giles and T. Kuhn (2015), London: Bloomsbury, pp. 184–188.

Brecht, B. (1952) 'Formal Problems Arising from the Theatre's New Content', in *Brecht on Theatre: The Development of an Aesthetic*, edited and translated by J. Willett (2001), London: Methuen, pp. 226–230.

Brecht, B. (1957a) 'Theatre for Pleasure or Theatre for Instruction', in *Brecht on Theatre*, edited by M. Silberman, S. Giles and T. Kuhn (2015), London: Bloomsbury, pp. 109–117.

Brecht, B. (1957b) 'On the Use of Music in an Epic Theatre', in *Brecht on Theatre*, edited by M. Silberman, S. Giles and T. Kuhn (2015), London: Bloomsbury, pp. 124–131.

Brecht, B. (1957c) '*Verfremdung* Effects in Chinese Acting', in *Brecht on Theatre*, edited by M. Silberman, S. Giles and T. Kuhn (2015), London: Bloomsbury, pp. 151–158.

Brecht, B. (1963) 'Two Essays on Unprofessional Acting', in *Brecht on Theatre: The Development of an Aesthetic*, edited and translated by J. Willett (2001), London: Methuen, pp. 148–153.

Brown, C.E. (2015) *Shakespeare and Psychoanalytic Theory*, London: Bloomsbury.

Butler, J. (1999) *Gender Trouble: Feminism and the Subversion of Identity*, London: Routledge.

Campbell, P. and Kear, A. (eds.) (2001) *Psychoanalysis and Performance*, London: Routledge.

Elam, K. (1980) *The Semiotics of Theatre and Drama*, London: Methuen.

Fischer-Lichte, E. (2008) *The Transformative Power of Performance: A New Aesthetics*, London: Routledge.

Freshwater, H. (2009) *Theatre and Audience*, Basingstoke: Palgrave Macmillan.

Freud, S. (1900) 'The Interpretation of Dreams', *The Standard Edition of the Complete Psychological Works of Sigmund Freud, Volume IV and V (1900)*, pp. ix–627, London: The Hogarth Press.

Freud, S. (1906) 'Psychopathic Characters on the Stage (1942 [1905 or 1906])', *The Standard Edition of the Complete Psychological Works of Sigmund Freud, Volume VII (1901–1905): A Case of Hysteria, Three Essays on Sexuality and Other Works*, pp. 303–310, London: The Hogarth Press.

Freud, S. (1907) 'Delusions and Dreams in Jensen's Gradiva', *The Standard Edition of the Complete Psychological Works of Sigmund Freud, Volume IX (1906–1908): Jensen's "Gradiva" and Other Works*, pp. 1–95, London: The Hogarth Press.

Freud, S. (1915) 'The Unconscious', *The Standard Edition of the Complete Psychological Works of Sigmund Freud, Volume XIV (1914–1916): On the History of the Psycho-Analytic Movement, Papers on Metapsychology and Other Works*, pp. 159–215, London: The Hogarth Press.

Freud, S. (1923) 'The Ego and the Id', *The Standard Edition of the Complete Psychological Works of Sigmund Freud, Volume XIX (1923–1925): The Ego and the Id and Other Works*, pp. 1–66, London: The Hogarth Press.

Freud, S. (1924) 'A Short Account of Psycho-Analysis (1924 [1923])', *The Standard Edition of the Complete Psychological Works of Sigmund Freud, Volume XIX (1923–1925): The Ego and the Id and Other Works*, pp. 189–210, London: The Hogarth Press.

Freud, S. (1925) 'An Autobiographical Study (1925 [1924])', *The Standard Edition of the Complete Psychological Works of Sigmund Freud, Volume XX (1925–1926): An Autobiographical Study, Inhibitions, Symptoms and Anxiety, Lay Analysis and Other Works*, pp. 1–74, London: The Hogarth Press.

Freud, S. (1926) 'The Question of Lay Analysis: Conversations with an Impartial Person', *The Standard Edition of the Complete Psychological Works of Sigmund Freud, Volume XX (1925–1926): An Autobiographical Study, Inhibitions, Symptoms and Anxiety, Lay Analysis and Other Works*, pp. 177–258, London: The Hogarth Press.

Freud, S. (1930) 'Civilization and Its Discontents', *The Standard Edition of the Complete Psychological Works of Sigmund Freud, Volume XXI (1927–1931): The Future of an Illusion, Civilization and Its Discontents and Other Works*, pp. 57–146, London: The Hogarth Press.

Gay, P. (2006) *Freud: A Life for Our Time*, New York/London: W. W. Norton.

Green, A. (1979) *The Tragic Effect: The Oedipus Complex in Tragedy*, translated by A. Sheridan, Cambridge: Cambridge University Press.

Irigaray, L. (1993) 'Psychoanalytic Theory: Another Look', in *This Sex Which Is Not One*, translated by C. Porter and C. Burke, New York: Cornell University Press, pp. 34–67.

McConachie, B. (2008) *Engaging Audiences: A Cognitive Approach to Spectating in the Theatre*, New York: Palgrave Macmillan.

Nuetzel, E.J. (1999) 'Acting and Enacting: A Case Study in the Evolution of Theatrical Performance', *Journal of Applied Psychoanalytic Studies*, vol. 1, no. 1, pp. 79–101.

Parker, S. (2014) *Bertolt Brecht: A Literary Life*, London: Bloomsbury.

Phelan, P. (1993) *Unmarked: The Politics of Performance*, London: Routledge.

Rousseau, J.-J. (1759) *Letter from M. Rousseau, of Geneva, to M. d'Alembert, of Paris, Concerning the Effects of Theatrical Entertainments on the Manners of Mankind*, translated from the French, London: Printed for J. Nourse at the Lamb opposite Katherine-Street in the Strand.

Veltruský, J. (1981) 'The Prague School Theory of Theater', *Poetics Today*, vol. 2, no. 3, pp. 225–235.

von Held, P. (2011) *Alienation and Theatricality: Diderot after Brecht*, Oxford: Legenda.

Chapter 2

Transference and *katharsis*, Freud to Aristotle

Introduction

Aristotle's theory of tragic *katharsis* has been 'the most celebrated concept in the entire field of literary criticism' (Golden, 1976: 437) and the subject of discussion and dispute at least since the rediscovery of the *Poetics* during the Renaissance and well into the twentieth century. Brecht took it as a point of reference for his condemnation of conventional theatre, in the context of his concern with the social and political function of this art. In doing so, he drew on the prevailing interpretation of *katharsis* as purgation without questioning its validity. This had profound implications for his theory of spectatorship: *katharsis* indicated a hypnotic experience supposed to induce the spectator into a passive state and to inhibit his capacity for critical distance. Accordingly, Brecht's assumptions excluded the possibility that unconscious dynamics may contribute productively to theatre reception. In this chapter, I will challenge the interpretation of *katharsis* which formed the basis of Brecht's understanding of spectatorship, and against which he framed his reform. By applying Freud's theory of transference to the analysis of *katharsis*, I will show that unconscious aspects of spectatorship are central to theatre reception.

Aristotle's theory of tragic *katharsis* is the most renowned pronouncement on spectatorship of all times. It is set forth in the *Poetics* (1449b24–28)[1] and it states that tragedy is 'a representation [*mimēsis*] of an action which is serious, complete [. . .] and through the arousal of pity and fear effecting the *katharsis* of such emotions'. Despite giving the impression of clarity, this dense definition has been the subject of controversies and of many attempts at explaining what it means (Halliwell, 1992). In particular, what Aristotle 'meant in claiming that tragedy produces a *katharsis*, is a question which has dominated western philosophy and literary criticism since the Renaissance' (Lear, 1988: 297). The debate has especially engaged with the question whether he meant purification of the emotions (their sublimation or perfection within the mind) or purification of the mind from the emotions (their discharge or abreaction from the mind) (Halliwell, 1992).

This second meaning has been the most accepted of the last hundred years, hence the tendency to translate *katharsis* as 'purgation'. Nevertheless the controversy has never abated and questions regarding the emotional versus the

This chapter is adapted from the following published article: Maria Grazia Turri, 'Transference and katharsis, Freud to Aristotle', *The International Journal of Psychoanalysis* 96.2 (Wiley, 2014) pp. 369–387.

intellectual nature of *katharsis*, its supposed or doubtful moral value, and the relative import of pity and fear, are still pending (Butcher, 1951; Golden, 1976; Fabbri, 2000). Some justification for translating *katharsis* as purgation is based on the hypothesis that Aristotle was probably the first author to apply the idea of *katharsis* to the theory of tragedy (Halliwell, 2002: 219) and had borrowed the term from the medical literature of his time (Jauss, 1982: 25). A passage in the *Politics* (1342a4–14),[2] where the philosopher is writing about *katharsis* in relation to the effects of music, affirms that in people whose soul is affected by strong emotions certain sacred melodies may induce a state of *katharsis* 'just as if they were receiving a medical treatment'.

On the other hand, the rendering of *katharsis* as sublimation or moral perfection has been very popular until the eighteenth century (Halliwell, 1986). But in the nineteenth century, there was the reaching of a general agreement to translating *katharsis* as purgation, albeit this has never been universally accepted (see for instance Golden, 1976). One of the most important contributions to this rendition was a book by Jakob Bernays,[3] originally published in German in 1857 (Lear, 1988: 297), which emphasized the medical origin of the term (Halliwell, 1992). Curiously, Bernays was Freud's wife's uncle, and Freud was well acquainted with his work (Stok, 2010). It seems therefore likely that Bernays's rendition of *katharsis* was relied on when his colleague Joseph Breuer suggested to Freud that they call the first psychoanalytic treatment the 'cathartic method' (Freud and Breuer, 1895). After it resided for many centuries in literary theory, Freud and Breuer returned the concept of *katharsis* back to medicine.

From their description of the cathartic method, it is evident that Freud and Breuer understand *katharsis* as purgation. Incidentally, we know that Freud was aware of Aristotle's theory at least as early as 1905 and that he translated *katharsis* as purging. In the opening paragraph of his introduction to *Psychopathic Characters on the Stage*, a work which he wrote in 1905 but was only published posthumously, he states:

> If, as has been assumed since the time of Aristotle, the purpose of drama is to arouse 'terror and pity' and so 'to purge the emotions' [. . .] the prime factor is unquestionably the process of getting rid of one's own emotions by 'blowing off steam'.
>
> (Freud, 1906: 305)

In this passage he is clearly translating *katharsis* with purging. Like it is for Brecht, '*Reinigung*' is the German word he employs.

After the formulation of the cathartic method, Freud further advanced his understanding of how psychoanalysis relieves psychic suffering, by discovering the phenomenon of transference. As I will show, examining the development of this psychoanalytic theory generates key insights into the question posed by literary scholars about Aristotelian *katharsis*: whether the effect on the emotions of psychoanalysis (for Freud) or theatre (in Aristotle) is about purging or rather perfecting them.

Aristotle's theory of *mimēsis* and tragic *katharsis*

When, in the *Politics* (1341b39–41), Aristotle mentions *katharsis* as one of the purposes of music, he anticipates that he will clarify its precise meaning in his future work of the *Poetics*, but unfortunately either this did not happen or we have lost the fragment containing his explanation. Moreover, there is a paucity of details in the *Politics* on which to rely in order to expand on Aristotle's ideas about the cathartic effect. The most interesting of these, is the relationship that Aristotle establishes between *katharsis* and *mimēsis*. In the *Poetics* (1449b24–28) Aristotle attributes the arousal of fear and pity to the mimetic character of tragedy, but he does not explain this any further. In the *Politics* (1340a12–14), talking about music, he indicates more clearly that he considers the mimetic quality of music responsible for the arousal of corresponding emotions: 'Furthermore, everyone who listens to representations [*mimēseon*] comes to have similar emotions, even apart from the rhythms and melodies of those representations'.

Applied to tragedy, this passage confirms that, in order to be subjected to *katharsis*, the emotions of fear and pity must be aroused through the *mimēsis* of tragic actions, thereby establishing that *mimēsis* is the necessary source of the cathartic effect. Understanding the meaning of *mimēsis* may therefore expand our knowledge of *katharsis*. In particular, there are three attributes of *mimēsis* which are relevant for my subsequent analysis of *katharsis* from a psychoanalytic perspective. First of all, despite being a polyseme, in the *Poetics mimēsis* has the more specific meaning of 'dramatic enactment'. Secondly, *mimēsis* is characteristic of human innate behaviour and it is a source of pleasure. Thirdly, it pertains to considerations about morality.

The concept of *mimēsis* figures in the pre-Socratic tradition (Halliwell, 2002: 15–16) and is amply used by Plato in a number of works and contexts, in connection with epistemology, ethics, psychology, politics and metaphysics (Halliwell, 2002: 24), and most notably in his critique of it in *Republic III* (386a–417b)[4] and *X* (595a–621d).[5] According to Aristotle all arts are forms of *mimēsis*. These include poetic arts such as tragedy, comedy, epic and dithyramb, as well as music and painting (*Poetics*, 1447a13–18, 1460b8–11). *Mimēsis* operates as a key factor that distinguishes artistic creation from other forms of human intellectual activity (*Poetics*, 1447b16–20). Within the arts, however, the denotative attributes of *mimēsis* are less clear. Like Aristotle, Plato applies *mimēsis* and its related terminology to both the musico-poetic and the visual arts (Halliwell, 2002: 24). Yet this is not univocally true and in *Republic III* (392c6–394b2) Plato refers to a restricted meaning of *mimēsis* as specifically denoting dramatic impersonation. As has been proposed, it is possible that *mimēsis* 'as popularly applied to poetry, was [. . .] suggested to the Greeks by those dramatic forms of poetry in which acting or recitation produced an impression allied to that of mimicry' (Butcher, 1951: 138).

In *Republic III* (392c6–394b2) the restricted meaning of *mimēsis* is specifically intended as personification in the dramatic art, i.e., the embodiment of a character, in opposition to narration [*diēgēsis*]. As explained through the words of Socrates, to whom Plato attributes the authority of his philosophy, poets can choose between two forms of telling their story: by narrating it or by talking as if they were the characters of the story. Tragedy and comedy are the paradigm of a poetic form entirely based on *mimēsis*, dithyrambs are based solely on narration, while epic poetry presents as a mixture of the two forms (*Republic III* 394b6–c5).

Aristotle himself refers to this restricted meaning in the *Poetics* (1460a5–11), when he suggests that one of the reasons why Homer is such a superior poet is that he lets his characters speak for themselves, and only rarely engages in narrative. Here Aristotle, somewhat contradicting what he had said elsewhere in the *Poetics*, distinguishes the poetic form based on narrative to the one based on *mimēsis*, granting *mimēsis* a denotation of the dramatic as opposed to other forms of poetic composition:

> Among Homer's many other laudable attributes is his grasp – unique among epic poets – of his status as poet. For the poet himself should speak as little as possible, since when he does so he is not engaging in mimesis. Now, other epic poets participate persistently, and engage in mimesis only to a limited extent and infrequently. But Homer, after a short preamble, at once brings onto stage a man, woman or some other figure.

It is often emphasized how Aristotle discounted dramatic representation as an essential component of tragedy, for example when, in the *Poetics* (1450b16–20), he wrote that spectacle is the least relevant component of tragedy, because the value of tragedy does not rest on its performance and should not depend on the art of the mask-maker or other visual effects. One should be wary however of maintaining that by doing so he ends up equating tragedy to a literary form. Other literary forms in Aristotle's times were represented through public readings and hence what the dramatic performance is here contrasted to is not likely to be a silent reading, but rather a recitation. What Aristotle may well be rejecting are the decorative elements of theatre (like masks, to which he specifically refers, or scenery) rather than the enacted rendition of text. Incidentally, the history of twentieth-century theatre does not lack masters who have similarly deplored the decorative aspects of theatrical spectacle, while emphasizing the importance of the actor's embodiment. Suffice to think of Grotowski (1975) and his formulation of 'the poor theatre'.

Talking about the composition of tragedy, Aristotle provides us with an important pointer to the central role of impersonation. Here there is an emphasis on enactment of gestures and arousal of affects with regards to the creative work of the poet (*Poetics*, 1455a22–34):

> So far as possible, the poet should even include gestures in the process of composition: for, assuming the same natural talent, the most convincing effect comes from those who actually put themselves in the emotions; and the truest impression of distress or anger is given by the person who experiences these feelings.

Within a far from unitary conception, *mimēsis* retains a specific area of meaning which refers to dramatic enactment. According to Plato, imitative poetry (*Republic*, 603c4–9) 'portrays men engaged in involuntary or voluntary actions, and as a result of their action believing that they have succeeded or failed, and either grieving or rejoicing in all these circumstances'. In the *Poetics* (1449b36–1450a3) Aristotle applies this definition to tragedy unquestioned:

> Since tragedy is a representation [*mimēsis*] of an action, and is enacted by agents, who must be characterized in both their character and their thought (for it is through these that we can also judge the qualities of their actions, and it is in their actions that all men either succeed or fail).

In the restricted meaning *mimēsis* stands for impersonation of a character in the dramatic form. More specifically, both Plato and Aristotle clarify that it refers to the impersonation of a character in action, whether such action is voluntary or not. Despite remaining influenced by the large semantic field of the word, in the *Poetics* Aristotle ultimately veers towards equating *mimēsis* with the impersonation of a dramatic role (Halliwell, 1986).

Whilst *mimēsis* refers to the activity of the artist, and especially of the actor, it is by no means confined to be a specialist skill; on the contrary, it is considered to be characteristic of human innate behaviour. According to Aristotle the peculiar character of artistic creativity, grounded as it is in *mimēsis*, derives from two natural causes: that man has got a natural propensity to *mimēsis*, expressed since childhood, and which facilitates his first steps in understanding; and that *mimēsis* is a universal source of pleasure for human beings (*Poetics*, 1448b4–10). Plato remarks on a related point, when in *Republic III* (395d1–3) he gets Socrates to ask: 'Or haven't you noticed that imitations, if they are practised much past youth, get established in the habits and nature of body, tones of voice, and mind?'. Here *mimēsis* is thought to be a natural predisposition that is responsible for acquired habits. The transformation of what is innate into what is acquired depends on the possibility to either foster or hinder the former in order to shape the latter. As the argument in *Republic III* (396a5-e2) goes, this should be precisely the call of a proper education, which will foster good habits through the *mimēsis* of good models and hinder bad habits through the abolition of *mimēsis* of bad models.

Both Plato and Aristotle recognize an intimate link between *mimēsis* and pleasure. A passage in the *Poetics* (1448b9–13) underlies the ability of artistic representation to attach an experience of pleasure to things that we would find painful to look at in their actual form, such as unattractive animals or cadavers. Similarly, in *Republic X* (605c10–605d5) Plato speaks of the compelling enjoyment which tragic *mimēsis* provides to its audience, inescapable even by the most virtuous philosophers:

> When even the best of us hear Homer, or some other tragic poet, imitating [*mimoumenou*] one of the heroes in a state of grief and making a long speech

> of lamentation, or even chanting and beating his breast, you know we enjoy it and give ourselves over to it. We suffer along with the hero and take his sufferings seriously. And we praise the one who affects us most in this way as a good poet.

A propensity to dramatic enactments is recognized as natural and innate, and part of human development. Even more significantly, it is considered the earliest form of meaning-making in human beings. Moreover, there is recognition that such enactment is a source of pleasure, so much so that it is difficult to evade its appeal. The attribute of being innate and the intimate link with pleasure seem, by implication, to grant *mimēsis* a certain compelling quality. Such quality will lead the two ancient philosophers to opposite conclusions with regard to the ethical value of *mimēsis*.

Both Aristotle and Plato are interested in the debate about the ethical qualities of *mimēsis*, although for Plato these considerations are imperative while Aristotle places pleasure above moral instruction as the chief aim of poetry (Butcher, 1951). Nevertheless moral considerations enter into the *Poetics*, and their subordination to pleasure may be more suggestive of a particular belief about the way theatre affects moral improvement than of a disregard for its relevance to the effect of tragedy. I will return to this point in Chapter 6.

As I have briefly anticipated above, in *Republic III* (396c5-e2) Plato distinguishes *mimēsis* on the basis of the objects that it sets out to represent, and proposes that it should be fostered for the good models but hindered for the bad ones. Yet in *Republic X* he proceeds to condemn *mimēsis* at all levels, regardless of whether the models it portrays are good or bad. Here *mimēsis* is described as a most dangerous impediment to the education of citizens, and it justifies the total banning of poets from the ideal city. Tragic *mimēsis*, which induces the audience to partake in the hero's grief, is seen as particularly dangerous and irrational, leading far from virtue and the truth (*Republic*, 604d-e). In the *Republic* (600e4–602c3), through Socrates's voice, Plato gives three justifications for the condemnation of *mimēsis*. At an ontological level, he engages in a long exposition which aims at showing how the mimetic objects are twice removed from the truth and hence of limited value to the ideal city. At a psychological level, he maintains that mimetic poetry promotes a resonance in the audience with feelings that belong to the irrational character to the detriment of reason (*Republic*, 604e1–5):

> Now, this element – the one that gets irritated – admits of much complex imitation; whereas the wise and quiet character, which always remains pretty much selfsame, is neither easy to imitate nor easy to understand when imitated – especially not at a festival where multifarious people are gathered together in theaters. For the experience being imitated is alien to them.

The poets, interested in pleasing their audience, will naturally choose to represent the irrational (*Republic*, 605a2–6), an argument which will be adopted by

Rousseau (1759: 15) in his invective against theatre in the *Lettre à D'Alembert*. Finally, on the moral plane, it is the tight link between *mimēsis* and pleasure which causes Socrates to bring the harshest charge (*Republic*, 605c6–8): 'But we haven't yet brought our chief charge against imitation [*mimēsis*]. For its power to corrupt all but a very few good people is surely an altogether terrible one'. Because of the compelling nature of *mimēsis*, which enchants even the best citizens into giving in to an irrational pleasure taken at the expense of reason, Plato ends up suggesting its global censure.

The Platonic overarching condemnation of *mimēsis* creates a precedent that cannot be ignored. Aristotle contradicts it by arguing that the link between pleasure and *mimēsis* constitutes one of the pillars on which the much-celebrated art of the poet stands, in no way alienating us from the truth. As he had explained in the *Politics* (1340a23–28), the pleasurable or painful emotions experienced at the view of the representation are akin to feelings that might arise in consequence of the view of its corresponding real object, rather providing a faithful surrogate for truth itself: 'Someone who is accustomed to feeling pain and pleasure in things that are likenesses is close to someone who reacts in the same manner to true things'.

In the last section of the *Poetics* (1461b26–62b15), Aristotle discusses the merit of tragedy as compared to that of epic poetry. Initially, he admits that if he were to judge the value of poetic genres on the basis of its spectators, tragedy would indeed be found to be the most vulgar, but he attributes the vulgar effects of tragic performances to the clumsy attitudes of actors (*Poetics*, 1461b33–62a8). Aristotle's assertion that actors may spoil the performance of any poetry, including epic recitations, does not need to imply an overarching condemnation of acting: the history of theatre does not lack practitioners who set off to reform acting departing from a condemnation of the form it has taken. According to the philosopher, there are nevertheless various reasons why tragedy is superior to epics, including its more condensed and unitary plot (*Poetics*, 1462b1–7). Yet its higher value is especially decreed by its superiority in attaining its aim (*Poetics*, 1462b12–15), which is to effect the *katharsis* of pity and fear. As we have seen, the cathartic effect is absolutely dependent on emotions having first been aroused through *mimēsis*. Because a work of art cannot be separated from its effects on its recipients, effects which constitute its intrinsic quality (Butcher, 1951), the greatest merit of *mimēsis* is indeed to enable *katharsis*.

Pity and fear

Pity and fear are the two emotions which are central and exclusive to Aristotle's definition of tragic *katharsis*. While the association of *katharsis* with tragedy was most likely Aristotle's original idea, the notion that pity and fear were central to the reception of serious poetry, including tragedy, was well established in ancient Greece, long before the *Poetics* (Halliwell, 2002: 218–219). Aristotle does not discuss pity and fear anywhere in the *Poetics*, but their description is to be found in the second book of the *Rhetoric*, where he examines a wide range of human emotions. In the section dedicated to it, fear [*phobos*] is described as 'a pain or disturbance due to a mental picture of some destructive or painful evil in the future [. . .] only if they appear not remote but so near as to be imminent' (*Rhetoric*, 1382a21–26).[6] Fear is about oneself, as Aristotle states: 'fear is felt by those who believe something to be likely to happen to them' (*Rhetoric*, 1382b34). In a later paragraph of the *Rhetoric*, pity [*eleos*] is defined as a 'feeling of pain caused by the sight of some evil, destructive or painful, which befalls one who does not deserve it, and which we might expect to befall ourselves or some friend of ours, and moreover to befall us soon' (*Rhetoric*, 1385b13–16). Pity, differently from fear, is felt about someone else, as long as the situation presents enough similarities to one's own conditions that one can imagine the same event might happen to him. Yet Aristotle specifies that when we witness a harmful event occurring to someone who is very close to us, such as one's son, fear rather than pity ensues:

> The people we pity are: those whom we know, if only they are not very closely related to us – in that case we feel about them as if we were in danger ourselves. For this reason Amasis did not weep, they say, at the sight of his son being led to death, but did weep when he saw his friend begging: the latter sight was pitiful, the former terrible, and the terrible is different from the pitiful.
>
> (*Rhetoric*, 1386a17–24)

There is hence a strict correlation between pity and fear and it is only when considering their reciprocity that Aristotle's notion of the effect of tragedy can be understood (Butcher, 1951). There are important similarities and differences between these two emotions. They both are forms of suffering in relation to some painful event, but while fear is aroused by the imagination of a personal direct involvement in a painful experience, pity is aroused by the vision of a painful experience happening to someone else. Importantly, Aristotle is quite specific in determining who this other person should be for pity to be aroused: close enough to our representation of the self, that one can imagine the same painful event could well be happening to him, but not too close to one's heart, like for instance one's son, in which case fear rather than pity ensues. There is an emphasis here on 'a rather delicate balance between psychological involvement and distance' (Halliwell, 2002: 215) that needs to take place in pity, an emphasis which is crucial to the understanding of tragic *katharsis*, as I will discuss later.

Freud's theory of psychoanalysis from the cathartic method to the transference

In 1895, a relatively unknown Viennese neurologist, Sigmund Freud, and his colleague Joseph Breuer, published *Studies on Hysteria*, a book which was later to become the foundational text of psychoanalysis, and a seminal work in its own right (Freud and Breuer, 1895). The book endeavoured to set forth a new scientific theory of hysteria, and for the first time, a clinical method to cure its symptoms. Freud and Breuer proposed that each hysterical symptom originates in a psychical trauma. The trauma originally provoked an emotional response (for example, disgust or anger) that for certain reasons could not be expressed at the time. Hence this emotional response was 'repressed', i.e., retained within the patient's unconscious psyche but lost to her awareness. The repressed affect (or strangulated, to use Freud's vivid metaphor) found a disguised way of expression through the body, in which it became a hysterical symptom (a paralysis, a spasm, the inability to speak, or any other).

Interlinked to the theory of the origin and meaning of hysterical symptoms was the discovery of how they could be cured. If it was a strangulated affect that caused the hysterical symptom in the first place, might the patient be liberated from the symptom if she eventually succeeded in giving expression to the affect? And how could this be obtained, given that the emotional response had at first been successfully repressed at the expense of the patient's health? Breuer discovered that through hypnosis, presumably because of the partly unconscious state that it produces, the patient could be induced to represent in her mind the original trauma and to re-experience it in its full emotional power. If under hypnosis the patient succeeded in expressing the repressed emotions, awakening from it she would be symptom-free. As Freud puts it:

> For we found, to our great surprise at first, that each individual hysterical symptom immediately and permanently disappeared when we had succeeded in bringing clearly to light the memory of the event by which it was provoked and in arousing its accompanying affect, and when the patient had described that event in the greatest possible detail and had put the affect into words.
>
> (Freud and Breuer, 1895: 6)

In the detailed exposition of several case studies, Freud and Breuer gave numerous clinical examples of such curative process. For the purpose of clarification, I will illustrate one example taken from the case study of Anna O., the first patient to enter the history of psychoanalysis (Freud and Breuer, 1895: 21–47). Anna was a young woman who had developed a plethora of hysterical symptoms around and following the death of her father, whom she had devotedly nursed for many months. One example of these was hydrophobia, a terror of drinking which resulted in Anna's refusal to drink any liquid. This had been so debilitating that she suffered a tormenting thirst and could only take fluids by eating large amounts of fruit. The theory went that, if Anna could bring to her mind the original trauma and give expression to the repressed affect, she would be able to abreact the feeling(s) associated with the trauma and hence be cured of the symptom. In fact, under hypnosis Anna recounted with disgust that once she had seen her English maid let her dog drink from a glass. Inhibited by the duties of politeness, Anna had repressed her feelings and not said anything. Under hypnosis, however, she could express the disgust and rage that she had then felt towards her maid. Giving expression to these feelings meant abreacting them, hence, freed from the strangulated affects, she asked for a glass of water, drank profusely and woke up from the hypnotic state with the glass at her lips. The symptom had been cured.[7]

At the point of publishing *Studies on Hysteria*, Freud was already dissatisfied with some aspects of the cathartic method. Part of his dissatisfaction stemmed from the fact that he found hypnosis short of his expectations to bring people to the arousal and expression of their repressed affects. But this is not the whole story. Not yet aware of the significance of his observations, he was also discovering transference. It is precisely in the last chapter of *Studies on Hysteria* dedicated to 'The Psychotherapy of Hysteria' (Freud and Breuer, 1895: 253–305) that transference gets its first mention. At this point Freud considered transference to be a mere impediment to treatment and he was certainly not aware of the weight that this discovery would carry for his future theory and practice. It took Freud another fifteen years to arrive at the conviction that the analysis of transference is the principal factor involved in the therapeutic action of psychoanalysis. In Freud's (1905: 117) own words: 'Transference, which seems ordained to be the greatest obstacle to psycho-analysis, becomes its most powerful ally'.

Freud (1905: 116) defined transference as a new version of impulses and fantasies that have been awakened in the patient and brought to her awareness by the analytic process, their peculiar characteristic being that they replace some person who was familiar to the patient with the person of the analyst. The repressed emotion which is being expressed is not an original emotion directed towards the therapist, but instead a reproduction of an emotion once directed towards a significant person in the patient's life. The critical difference with the cathartic method is that the representation and expression of the repressed emotion is here achieved not in the mind of the patient, but in a communicative re-enactment with the therapist. Freud (1909) gave a significant example of his discovery of the transference as an important therapeutic tool in the famous case study of the Rat Man. The Rat Man was a young man so nicknamed after one of his most characteristic obsessional thoughts: that his deceased father might suffer a horrid torture implying live rats being made to enter the anus of the victim. The obsessive thought had first entered the Rat Man's mind one day when a fellow military captain had mentioned the horrible torture during a conversation; the Rat Man had instantly felt a sense of disgust, but immediately afterwards he had imagined his father as the victim of the torture and the thought had since represented itself to his mind in an obsessive manner. This symptom was the more tormenting for the Rat Man, as it seemed to have first been generated as a sadistic fancy, but this supposition was cruelly at variance with the Rat Man's affectionate and devoted feelings for his father. These were the only feelings he could recognize in himself ever to have felt towards his parent.

In the course of therapy, an episode belonging to the Rat Man's childhood was unveiled. His mother had told the Rat Man that when he was about three years old, he had been beaten by his father for having bit someone. To this he had rebelled so furiously, hurling insulting words at his assailant, that his father had stopped in astonishment and declared, 'The child will either be a great man or a great criminal!' (Freud, 1909: 265). The Rat Man had no personal recollection of such a memorable story. Not doubting the truth of his mother's words, he superficially conceded to Freud that this early scene bore some evidence of anger and rancour towards his father. Nevertheless his estrangement from any hostile feelings remained unshakeable, until when, and only when, these feelings eventually emerged in the transference. Some time after the memory was reported in analysis, insults towards Freud made their appearance in the Rat Man's associations, alongside impulses to punch Freud during the sessions, impulses that compelled the patient to walk around the room in an attempt to keep them at bay. The Rat Man was ashamed as he could not establish what might be the reason for his overbearing hostility towards his analyst. Prepared by observations that he had conducted with other patients but not taken yet to their full consequences, Freud attributed this apparently nonsensical situation to the transference. According to his new theoretical view of the transference, the Rat Man's hostile feelings for his analyst were the representation of the long-buried hostility for his father. The transference was the necessary medium for the re-experiencing of affects otherwise inaccessible, because only the actual re-experiencing of the hostile feelings could defeat the Rat Man's estrangement from them.

The Rat Man's expressions of hostility towards his person gave Freud the necessary foundation on which to build his interpretation of the Rat Man's repressed hostility for his father. Beforehand, Freud's suggestions that the patient's obsessions might have been generated by some unconscious rancour for his parent had always met with incredulity and denial. But once the transference had allowed the arousal of the repressed feelings, these were put at the disposal of analysis. Freud's interpretation assigned the significance of these emotions to the patient's past relationship with his father. Through this procedure, the Rat Man finally reached an awareness of the existence within his mind of these powerful and previously repressed emotions. Brought to consciousness, the feelings were finally deprived of their despotic ascendancy on the mind and the Rat Man could walk away freed of his horrific obsessions. The psychoanalytic treatment had proved successful.

Transference re-enactment and transference analysis

According to Freud (1912), the merit of the transference is to allow the representation of an emotion which would otherwise remain repressed and manifest itself as a symptom impinging on the patient's health. Here Freud does not speak any longer purely of hysterical symptoms, but of any kind of symptoms, for example an obsession in the case of the Rat Man. Freud (1914: 150) understands this representation as a re-enactment: 'the patient does not *remember* anything of what he has forgotten and repressed, but *acts* it out. He reproduces it not as a memory but as an action; he *repeats* it, without, of course, knowing that he is repeating it'. This re-enactment of repressed emotions (for example, the anger for the father in the Rat Man's case) is compelling and while it may get activated in any current situation which the patient finds himself in, it becomes particularly prominent in the course of the analytic treatment.

> As long as the patient is in the treatment he cannot escape from this compulsion to repeat; and in the end we understand that this is his way of remembering. [. . .] We must be prepared to find, therefore, that the patient yields to the compulsion to repeat [. . .] not only in his personal attitude to his doctor but also in every other activity and relationship which may occupy his life at the time.
>
> (Freud, 1914: 150–151)

But for the scope of the successful outcome of the analytic treatment, the transference as means of representation and expression of the repressed has only accomplished half of its task, and a dangerous albeit necessary half. The response of the analyst to the re-enactment is crucial to determining the outcome of the transference cure.

In a paper dedicated to the erotic transference and its management, Freud (1915) warned against two equally detrimental and opposite tactics in which the analyst might respond to the transference: inviting the patient to repress her erotic longings for the analyst, or giving in to the temptation of satisfying them. It is in the transference that the patient mostly looks for surrogate satisfaction of her repressed desires and it is on this ground that the physician must leave her 'with unfulfilled wishes in abundance' (Freud, 1919: 164). Especially the risk of responding by what in psychoanalytic jargon has become known as 'acting in' on the part of the analyst represents the greatest hindrance for the progress of analysis. Again on the specific case of erotic transference, Freud (1915: 166) writes:

> If the patient's advances were returned it would be a great triumph for her, but a complete defeat for the treatment. She would have succeeded [. . .] in acting out, in repeating in real life, what she ought only to have remembered, to have reproduced as psychical material and to have kept within the sphere of psychical events.

Although Freud is here specifically talking about erotic transference, these reflections can be generalized to all transference situations.

In order for the re-enactment in the transference to effect a curative process, the analyst needs to engage in

> a perpetual struggle with his patient to keep in the psychical sphere all the impulses which the patient would like to direct into the motor sphere; and he celebrates it as a triumph for the treatment if he can bring it about that something that the patient wishes to discharge in action is disposed of through the work of remembering.
>
> (Freud, 1914: 153)

By avoiding 'acting in', the analyst allows the patient to recognize that the repressed affect belonged to a past relationship between him and another person: 'We soon perceive that the transference is itself only a piece of repetition, and that the repetition is a transference of the forgotten past' (Freud, 1914: 151). It is such recognition, given through an analytic interpretation, which creates a healthy distance to be put between the emotion itself and the patient today.

It is possible to illustrate the two facets of the transference by returning to the example of the Rat Man's obsession (Freud, 1909). When the Rat Man expressed his aggressive impulses towards Freud, he was going through the re-enactment phase of the transference, the one in which he was finally re-experiencing a long-repressed affect (anger and hostility). If Freud had chosen to ignore these impulses, or dismiss them as senseless, he would have allied himself with the repressing forces. If Freud had instead been frightened or critical of them, he would have 'acted in', repeating the original response that the Rat Man's father had given to the Rat Man's anger, when he stopped beating the child and predicted he might be a genius or a criminal, showing a mixture of astonishment and concern about his son's strong, angry feelings. In both these cases, the re-expression of feelings would have led to the reinforcement of their repression. Instead, by recognizing the feelings as part of the transference, the analyst can foster awareness of them in the patient. Ultimately, through the tool of interpretation, the analyst formulates and communicates to the patient his recognition of the feelings as part of the transference and their attribution to their original situation. By doing so, he is hoping to make conscious what was unconscious, hence working against repression. When repression is eventually overcome, the patient is freed from the symptom that represented the disguised expression of the repressed emotions.

The final outcome of the analysis of transference compares to the one that Freud had theorized for the cathartic method, namely overcoming of repression and bringing unconscious emotions into the patient's awareness; however, not only has the technique changed, but also the related theory. In the cathartic method it was the discharge from the mind of aroused affects which was taken as the curative factor: here the emotions were presumed to be removed from the mind. In the transference, instead, it is the interpretation of the aroused affects as belonging to a past relationship which effects the cure by conferring them meaning. Here the emotions are presumed to be processed within the mind.

Repetition-compulsion – beyond the pleasure principle

In a seminal paper with the suggestive title *Beyond the Pleasure Principle*, Freud (1920) turns to explore the significance of the compulsion to repeat seen in the re-enactment phase of transference. He explains that he has also encountered this phenomenon in the way trauma is represented in patients' dreams over and over again, and in some instances of children's play. What Freud sets out to understand is why it appears that the repetition-compulsion associated with a traumatic experience takes precedence over the striving for its pleasurable resolution. The importance of this question lies in the fact that it challenges the idea Freud (1911) held up to this point that the fundamentals of psychic life are organized by the pleasure and the reality principles, and that both of them, either directly or indirectly, have as their final aim the reaching of a state of pleasure.

In order to illustrate this point, Freud (1920) gives a detailed observation of a game that his grandson has been engaging with at the age of one and half. The little boy, who was very obedient and showed little protest at times when his mother would leave him for a few hours, had a habit of throwing objects into a corner of his room while vocalising a long drawn-out 'o-o-o-o', which Freud could establish stood for the German word '*fort*', which means 'gone'. The child used to repeat this game untiringly, and without displaying any evident pleasure in it. However at times, but much less frequently, he also played a variant of the game, when a reel attached to a string was first thrown out of sight, coupled with the expressive 'o-o-o-o', but subsequently pulled back to its reappearance, which was accompanied instead by a joyful '*da*' [there]. Freud interprets the game as a re-enactment of the little boy's feelings about his mother leaving him. While the boy refrains from protesting at his beloved mother's departure, he stages her disappearance over and over by representing it with the throwing away of the objects. Interestingly, while this act of disappearance is staged relentlessly, the second act of making the object return is only rarely performed, despite being evidently the pleasurable part of the game and despite it representing what would seem to be the most desirable aim, the mother's return.

If one cannot maintain that the act of throwing away the object is acted out by the child as a preliminary to the enactment of the joyful satisfaction of getting it back, which alternative explanation can be given and how does it fit with the supremacy of the pleasure principle in Freud's theory of the psyche? Freud eventually comes to the conclusion (corroborated by a number of other observations) that there must be a principle of psychic functioning which lies 'beyond the pleasure principle'. In Freud's (1920: 16) words:

> one gets an impression that the child turned his experience into a game for another motive. At the outset he was in a *passive* situation – he was overpowered by the experience; but, by repeating it, unpleasurable though it was, as a game, he took on an *active* part. These efforts might be put down to an instinct for mastery that was acting independently of whether the memory was in itself pleasurable or not.

Freud's conclusion is that beyond the pleasure principle, at a more fundamental level, the psyche engages in repetition-compulsion as the groundwork for all psychic processes. The repetition-compulsion which manifests itself in the transference re-enactment turns out to be the most fundamental phenomenon of psychic life. In reference to children's play, Freud (1920: 17) states that the centrality of such phenomenon implies that 'that there is no need to assume the existence of a special imitative instinct in order to provide a motive for play'. In other words, if from a popular view, the motive of play may have been seen as imitation, from Freud's new perspective it may be regarded as the instinct for mastery of psychic pain through repetition-compulsion.

An interpretation of tragic *katharsis* as transference dynamic

It is perhaps because *katharsis* talks about the way our mind deals with emotions and aims at explaining 'the relationship between the soul and the body' (Fabbri, 2000) that the introduction of the concept of *katharsis* from the realm of medicine to that of poetics operated by Aristotle (Jauss, 1982: 25) has ignited our imagination for more than two thousand years. When Freud and Breuer (1895) used the term 'cathartic method' to describe their new cure of hysterical symptoms, they borrowed the term *katharsis* from Aristotle's *Poetics* or rather from the ample referencing that the term had long enjoyed. Freud's journey, from the cathartic method to the transference, hints at Freud's struggle with the question of how a therapeutic technique can help our psyche process emotions: does psychoanalysis act as a purging effect (the cathartic cure) by releasing entangled emotions or, in a more complex but also finer way, does it promote the attribution of meaning to emotions causing their transformation from a compelling, irrational and unconscious status to a reflective and conscious one? It is of course the second explanation which will be gradually unveiled and brought to the fore by the theory of transference. There is a striking parallel here with the debate around the Aristotelian meaning of katharsis, urging a comparison between tragic katharsis and transference.

According to Aristotle, *katharsis* is possible only after the emotions of fear and pity have been aroused by *mimēsis*. Although *mimēsis* is a complex concept, in the *Poetics* Aristotle mainly refers to it as meaning dramatic enactment. This is a first point of correspondence with the transference phenomenon: *mimēsis* intended as dramatic enactment functions for the spectator like re-enactment in the transference functions for the patient, in as far as both *katharsis* and the analysis of transference are possible only following, respectively, the arousal of emotions through *mimēsis* or through transference re-enactments. Moreover, the relation between *mimēsis* and transference re-enactment runs even deeper in as far as it is through an action that both processes allow emotions to be experienced, or more precisely through a surrogate action. In the case of theatre reception, the surrogate action is the representation of the tragic actions by the performers, while, in the case of transference, it is the patient's re-enactment with the analyst. Transference re-enactments are forms of repetition-compulsion and repetition-compulsion enables the representation of repressed emotions in action. In the example of the young child throwing away objects over and over again, this surrogate action is performed to represent the painful experience of his mother leaving him (Freud, 1920). In the transference, the surrogate action consists of the re-enactment of an emotional dynamic between patient and analyst, like the expressions of anger that the Rat Man enacted towards Freud (Freud, 1909). Such a phenomenon is the departing point of analysis, what enables the repressed emotions to be aroused so that they can be subjected to the analytic work. Like *mimēsis* enables *katharsis*, so transference re-enactments enable psychoanalysis.

Both *mimēsis* and transference re-enactments (intended as a form of repetition-compulsion) are fundamental phenomena of psychic life and have an intimate link with pleasure. According to both Aristotle and Plato, *mimēsis* is an innate principle of psychic development. Aristotle attributes to it the ability to facilitate a child's first steps in understanding, while Plato identifies it as the natural predisposition to the formation of habits. Freud believes that repetition-compulsion is an innate and primary psychic process which gets activated each time that a repressed emotional experience needs to be made sense of, and in this way it equates, in psychoanalysis, to the birth of any understanding. In as far as repetition-compulsion is at the basis of unconscious representations of emotional dynamics (for example the Rat Man's anger for his father), it also represents the matrix of psychological 'habits', for example the tendency of a man like the Rat Man to re-enact anger towards surrogate figures who come to represent his father, like Freud in the transference or other significant people in his present life. Freud's case study talks of the Rat Man's aggressive fantasies towards his fiancée and other significant persons in his life, a further symptom of his repressed emotions.

Both Plato and Aristotle recognize an intimate link between *mimēsis* and pleasure. For Plato, *mimēsis* has a compelling quality, the paradigmatic example being the virtuous philosopher giving himself over to the enjoyment of tragic representations of grief, even if rationally he recognizes them as inappropriate or undesirable. Here the parallel with repetition-compulsion lies in the compelling quality of the arousal of emotions, which, despite appearing irrational, can take over even the most rational mind. Although *mimēsis* does not need to be identified solely with the irrational, whilst it is the case for the obligatory association between repetition-compulsion and the unconscious, Plato is clearly inclined to link *mimēsis* with lack of reason, one of the main motives for its condemnation. For Aristotle, the link between *mimēsis* and pleasure is proved by the attraction which mimetic objects, by which he means works of art, exert on all human beings. He further specifies that the surrogate nature of *mimēsis*, as realized in all art, including but not limited to tragedy, allows us to feel pleasure in situations when looking at the real objects in their actual form, such as unattractive animals or cadavers, would prove painful.

The link between repetition-compulsion and pleasure, a complex one, reveals some correspondence with Aristotle's insights into *mimēsis*. Freud's (1911) first thorough model of the mind postulated the pleasure principle as the basic principle of psychic life. However, Freud (1920) later found out that what he had imagined to be the ultimate drive of any human psychic activity, namely the search for pleasure, gets outclassed by the psychic mechanism of repetition-compulsion, which dictates psychic functioning 'beyond the pleasure principle'. In the psychoanalytic experience of the Rat Man, the child's murderous anger towards his father, memorable for the family history but personally forgotten by its protagonist because intolerably painful, is compelled to get re-expressed in the Rat Man's adult obsessions (Freud, 1909). The Rat Man's childhood experience of his father's beating evoked powerful feelings of anger and a thirst for revenge, a desire of putting his father in the position of being the victim. His obsession of rats entering his father's anus is the representation of an action in which the Rat Man, with sadistic pleasure, witnesses (or rather engineers in unconscious fantasy) the victimization of his father. Repressed emotions are so powerful that they beguile the unconscious mind into an incessant repetition where pleasure and displeasure are interlinked and the mastering of pain is equated to a fundamental experience of pleasure.

In his first formulation of the theory of repetition-compulsion, while discussing its links with the pleasure principle, Freud (1920: 17) inserted a short reflection hinting at the implications of his new theory for the understanding of theatre reception.

> Finally, a reminder may be added that the artistic play and artistic imitation carried out by adults, which, unlike children's, are aimed at an audience, do not spare the spectators (for instance, in tragedy) the most painful experiences and can yet be felt by them as highly enjoyable. This is convincing proof that [. . .] there are ways and means enough of making what is in itself unpleasurable into a subject to be recollected and worked over in the mind.

In this passage Freud comes closest to affirming that the principle of repetition-compulsion lies at the basis of the value of spectatorship. However, he does not further elaborate on this point neither in this nor in future works.

The link that both *mimēsis* and re-enactment have with pleasure poses the question, in the classical debate as well as in Freud, of their ethical value. Earlier I have illustrated the controversy between Plato and Aristotle: *mimēsis* can be seen as dangerous (Plato) in as far as it promotes in the audience the arousal of feelings which belong to the irrational character to the detriment of reason; but it is a precious and valuable process (Aristotle) in as far as it allows the arousal of truthful emotions and it constitutes the basis for *katharsis*. For Freud the value of re-enactment as a surrogate of a repressed emotional experience consists in putting unconscious unprocessed material at the disposal of analysis, which, if conducted properly, will lead to the proposition 'Where id was, there ego shall be', that is the transformation of repressed unconscious emotions into conscious thoughts (Freud, 1933: 80). Yet any re-enactment, being a surrogate of a true experience, is both truthful and deceitful. It is a self-deceit in as far as the hysterical patient believes herself to be in love with her analyst or the Rat Man believes himself angry with Freud. If such re-enactments, with their compelling quality, manage to find an actualization without being subject to the analytic work, they represent dangerous distortions of the truth, which lead to the replication of a past trauma. Instead, if they come to be helpfully seized as bedrock for the analytic work, they represent the golden road to the truth.

Tragic katharsis *as transference dynamic*

The existence of a parallel dynamic between re-enactment and analysis in transference and *mimēsis* and *katharsis* in spectatorship can help answer the question of what *katharsis* means – purgation or perfection? – and hence what might be the effect of the theatrical experience on the spectator's emotions. Here it is useful to return to the other central point for the interpretation of Aristotle's theory of tragic *katharsis*: the specific reference to the emotions of pity and fear, which are exclusive to the definition of tragic *katharsis*. According to Aristotle, both these emotions are forms of suffering but, while fear is self-referential, pity implies suffering for someone similar enough to oneself that one could imagine being this other person, but not so close to one's heart that fear instead would be aroused. There is a gap between fear and pity, which emphasizes the measure of one's 'distance' between the self and the representation of another as a possible self. For the scope of a psychoanalytic interpretation of tragic *katharsis*, such a measure of distance is crucial. Returning for a moment to reflect on transference, what determines its therapeutic effect is the ability to let repressed affects be aroused and subsequently analyzed. Both the arousal and the analysis are essential to the therapeutic process, as there would be no emotions available for analysis unless they were first aroused and experienced; but most importantly the arousal not followed by analysis would be anti-therapeutic. The transference re-enactment is therefore a double-edged sword: dangerous trigger to the repetition of traumatic experiences or unique opportunity for the overcoming of compelling dynamics, which, lifted from the recesses of the unconscious, can be subjected to reflection and understanding. It is the analysis of transference which puts the unconscious dynamic under the scrutiny of reason. Such scrutiny is based on the ability of the analyst to maintain a distancing and observing posture towards the re-enactment: interested in it enough but able to see it for what it is, a surrogate of truth.

By interpreting the re-enacted emotion as alive in the present, but its meaning belonging to the patient's past, the analyst achieves a regulation of distance between the patient and his previously repressed emotion(s), allowing a 'working through' from the unconscious to the conscious. Similarly, *mimēsis* is the dramatic enactment which facilitates the spectator's emotional participation in the tragic events in full identification with the character(s), as if he were imagining himself personally involved in the tragic actions. At the same time, suggests Aristotle, tragedy also promotes a distancing effect between the spectator and the emotions of the character(s), as if his involvement in the painful experience compares to that of a sympathetic witness. *Katharsis* is hence neither an immersive emotional identification with the hero which results in a release of tension, a sort of purgation of the emotions, nor a detached or rational re-elaboration of the meaning of emotions from an observing perspective; it is instead the fruitful dynamic between close emotional identification and sympathetic detachment which represents the quintessential meaning of tragic *katharsis*.

Brecht's reading of Aristotelian *katharsis* as a hypnotic experience reducing the spectator to a passive sufferer of the character's emotions may therefore be justified only so far as spectatorship is believed to be limited to the experience of 'fear', that is, of an unconscious emotional identification that compels the spectator to feel himself to be the character. That is what Brecht (1951: 184) derogatorily calls 'the empathy operation'. As transference shows, and as Plato's concerns about *mimēsis* illustrate, unconscious emotional identification amounts to repetition-compulsion, a re-enactment of repressed emotions which can lead to further re-traumatization. On the other hand, repetition-compulsion is the groundwork for psychic development, and re-enactments are the essential foundation of self-awareness, provided that a transition from the unconscious to the conscious is achieved. By dismissing *katharsis* as a passive and undesirable experience, Brecht is overlooking the potential merit of empathy in relation to one's capability for insight and self-understanding.

In actual fact, admitting that the spectator's unconscious emotional identification with the character in fear corresponds to the re-experiencing of the spectator's own repressed emotions, then the reflective distancing prompted by pity is equivalent to a form of self-analysis, whereby the spectator, having identified closely with the character's emotions through *mimēsis*, is led to take a meta-position with reference to himself, a look of sympathy which allows him to become aware of his repressed emotions through the representation of a character as a possible self. Reason can thus talk to feeling, in a relationship of mutual psychic growth which overtakes the split between compulsive irrationality and a detached and repressive rationality. Accordingly, the transference dynamic between spectator and character turns spectatorship into an opportunity for psychic integration which favours the processing of unconscious emotions. Thus it may leave us unsurprised why Aristotle gave tragedy such a pre-eminence above all poetic arts.

Notes

1 All quotations from Aristotle's *Poetics* are from: Aristotle, *The Poetics of Aristotle*, translation and commentary by S. Halliwell (London: Duckworth, 1987).
2 All quotations from Aristotle's *Politics* are from: Aristotle, *Politics, Books VII and VIII*, translation and commentary by R. Kraut (Oxford: Clarendon Press, 1997).
3 Jakob Bernays, *Zwei Abhandlungen über die aristotelische Theorie des Drama* (Berlin: W. Hertz, 1880). A chapter of this book has been translated as 'Aristotle on the Effects of Tragedy' by Jonathan and Jennifer Barnes in: *Articles on Aristotle*. Vol. 4 (J. Barnes, M. Schofield & R. Sorabji eds., London, 1979).
4 All quotations from Plato's *Republic* except for *Republic X* are from: Plato, *Republic*, translated from the New Standard Greek Text, and introduction by C. D. C. Reeve (Indianapolis/Cambridge: Hackett Publishing Company, 2004).
5 All quotations from Plato's *Republic X* are from: Plato, *Plato: Republic 10*, translation and commentary by S. Halliwell (Warminster: Aris and Phillips, 1988).
6 All quotations from Aristotle's *Rhetoric* are from: Aristotle, *The Rhetoric and the Poetics of Aristotle*, translated by W. R. Roberts (New York: Random House, 1954).
7 At this very early stage of psychoanalysis, the Oedipus complex had yet to be discovered. Although it is reasonable to hypothesize that Freud would have formulated the development of hysteria in Anna O. as linked to her unresolved Oedipus complex for her dying father, and the anxieties and conflicts that this would imply, Freud and Breuer's present theory could not contemplate this occurrence. Given that Freud will radically

modify his account of the curative factors in psychoanalysis, the relevance of the case history of Anna O. lies in illustrating Freud's view of the cathartic effect, as he conceived it in this first phase of his research into the unconscious.

Bibliography

Aristotle (1954) *The Rhetoric and the Poetics of Aristotle*, translated by W.R. Roberts, New York: Random House.

Aristotle (1987) *The Poetics of Aristotle*, translation and commentary by S. Halliwell, London: Duckworth.

Aristotle (1997) *Politics, Books VII and VIII*, translation and commentary by R. Kraut, Oxford: Clarendon Press.

Brecht, B. (1951) 'Short Description of a New Technique of Acting That Produces a *Verfremdung* Effect', in *Brecht on Theatre*, edited by M. Silberman, S. Giles and T. Kuhn (2015), London: Bloomsbury, pp. 184–188.

Butcher, S.H. (1951) *Aristotle's Theory of Poetry and Fine Art*, New York: Dover Publications.

Fabbri, P. (2000) 'Catharsis: Again?', in *AA.VV., Semiotic Efficacity and the Effectiveness of the Text*, S. Marino: Breplos, [Online], Available: http://www.paolofabbri.it/saggi/catharsis.html

Freud, S. (1905) 'Fragment of an Analysis of a Case of Hysteria (1905 [1901])', *The Standard Edition of the Complete Psychological Works of Sigmund Freud, Volume VII (1901–1905): A Case of Hysteria, Three Essays on Sexuality and Other Works*, pp. 1–122, London: The Hogarth Press.

Freud, S. (1906) 'Psychopathic Characters on the Stage (1942 [1905 or 1906])', *The Standard Edition of the Complete Psychological Works of Sigmund Freud, Volume VII (1901–1905): A Case of Hysteria, Three Essays on Sexuality and Other Works*, pp. 303–310, London: The Hogarth Press.

Freud, S. (1909) 'Notes Upon a Case of Obsessional Neurosis', *The Standard Edition of the Complete Psychological Works of Sigmund Freud, Volume X (1909): Two Case Histories: "Little Hans" and the "Rat Man"*, pp. 151–318, London: The Hogarth Press.

Freud, S. (1911) 'Formulations on the Two Principles of Mental Functioning', *The Standard Edition of the Complete Psychological Works of Sigmund Freud, Volume XII (1911–1913): The Case of Schreber, Papers on Technique and Other Works*, pp. 213–226, London: The Hogarth Press.

Freud, S. (1912) 'The Dynamics of Transference', *The Standard Edition of the Complete Psychological Works of Sigmund Freud, Volume XII (1911–1913): The Case of Schreber, Papers on Technique and Other Works*, pp. 97–108, London: The Hogarth Press.

Freud, S. (1914) 'Remembering, Repeating and Working-Through (Further Recommendations on the Technique of Psycho-Analysis II)', *The Standard Edition of the Complete Psychological Works of Sigmund Freud, Volume XII (1911–1913): The Case of Schreber, Papers on Technique and Other Works*, pp. 145–156, London: The Hogarth Press.

Freud, S. (1915) 'Observations on Transference-Love (Further Recommendations on the Technique of Psycho-Analysis III)', *The Standard Edition of the Complete Psychological Works of Sigmund Freud, Volume XII (1911–1913): The Case of Schreber, Papers on Technique and Other Works*, pp. 157–171, London: The Hogarth Press.

Freud, S. (1919) 'Lines of Advance in Psycho-Analytic Therapy', *The Standard Edition of the Complete Psychological Works of Sigmund Freud, Volume XVII (1917–1919): An Infantile Neurosis and Other Works*, pp. 157–168, London: The Hogarth Press.

Freud, S. (1920) 'Beyond the Pleasure Principle', *The Standard Edition of the Complete Psychological Works of Sigmund Freud, Volume XVIII (1920–1922): Beyond the Pleasure Principle, Group Psychology and Other Works*, pp. 1–64, London: The Hogarth Press.

Freud, S. (1933) 'New Introductory Lectures on Psycho-Analysis (1933 [1932])', *The Standard Edition of the Complete Psychological Works of Sigmund Freud, Volume XXII (1932–1936): New Introductory Lectures on Psycho-Analysis and Other Works*, pp. 3–182, London: The Hogarth Press.

Freud, S. and Breuer, J. (1895) *Studies on Hysteria: The Standard Edition of the Complete Psychological Works of Sigmund Freud, Volume II (1893–1895)*, London: The Hogarth Press.

Golden, L. (1976) 'The Clarification Theory of "Katharsis" ', *Hermes*, vol. 104, pp. 437–458.

Grotowski, J. (1975) *Towards a Poor Theatre*, edited by E. Barba, London: Methuen.

Halliwell, S. (1986) *Aristotle's Poetics*, London: Duckworth.

Halliwell, S. (1992) 'Catharsis', in *A Companion to Aesthetics*, edited by D.E. Cooper, Oxford: Blackwell, pp. 61–63.

Halliwell, S. (2002) *The Aesthetics of Mimesis: Ancient Texts and Modern Problems*, Princeton: Princeton University Press.

Jauss, H.R. (1982) *Aesthetic Experience and Literary Hermeneutics*, Minneapolis: University of Minnesota Press.

Lear, J. (1988) 'Katharsis', *Phronesis*, vol. 33, no. 3, pp. 297–326.

Plato (1988) *Plato: Republic 10*, translation and commentary by S. Halliwell, Warminster: Aris and Phillips.

Plato (2004) *Republic*, translated from the New Standard Greek Text, and introduction by C.D.C. Reeve, Indianapolis/Cambridge: Hackett Publishing Company.

Rousseau, J.-J. (1759) *Letter from M. Rousseau, of Geneva, to M. d'Alembert, of Paris, Concerning the Effects of Theatrical Entertainments on the Manners of Mankind*, translated from the French, London: Printed for J. Nourse at the Lamb opposite Katherine-Street in the Strand.

Stok, F. (2010) 'Psychology', in *A Companion to the Classical Tradition*, edited by C.W. Callendorf, Oxford: Wiley, pp. 355–370.

Chapter 3

The *Paradoxe* inside out

Introduction

In the previous chapter I focused on the analysis of spectatorship with particular reference to Aristotle's definition of tragic *katharsis*. By interpreting *katharsis* as transference dynamic between spectator and character, I suggested that spectatorship may imply, at an unconscious level, a form of self-analysis. The spectator's emotional identification with the character through *mimēsis* is a vehicle for the arousal of his unprocessed emotions, repressed within his unconscious. *Katharsis* promotes a shift in the spectator's mind from close identification to taking a sympathetic stance towards the character's emotions, through which the spectator's unconscious emotions are released from the mechanism of repression and become available for conscious thought, engendering self-awareness. In psychoanalysis, the transference dynamic arises within the emotional relationship between the patient and the analyst, and it is the analyst's response to the patient which promotes the transformation of the re-enactment into self-awareness. Only when the analyst can maintain the patient's unconscious affects within the psychic sphere, resisting 'acting in' and conveying their meaning through an interpretation, the submission of the patient to the compulsion to repeat will have an opportunity to be worked through into self-reflection and psychic development.

When Brecht took issue against *katharsis*, interpreting it as the spectator's subjugation to passive emotional identification with the character and disavowal of his critical distance, he also suggested that it is the actor and her own identification with the character that are the means through which the spectator's hypnotic submission is realized. Brecht typifies the essence of spectatorship as 'a mirroring relation between actor and spectator' (von Held, 2011: 43) suggesting a tight correspondence between conscious and unconscious acting techniques and their conscious or unconscious (hypnotic, in Brecht's terms) effects on the audience. Brecht's promotion of a new way of acting based on the *Verfremdungseffekt* is squarely founded upon his belief that the actor's interpretation of her character, and particularly the way she approaches the character's emotions, are a clue to the spectator's emotional and intellectual response. When the actor yields to feeling the character's emotions, the spectator will passively resonate with those same emotions, hypnotized into a state of thoughtless sentimentality. In order to preclude this harmful effect on the audience, the actor must renounce any feelings and assume an attitude of intellectual curiosity towards the character's emotions, so that the spectator will, by implication, mirror her approach. The spectator of the epic theatre is deprived of the empathic experience grounded in unconscious reverberation, in order that he can be supplied with an intellectual experience based on emulating the actor's detached observation of her character, ultimately engaging his reason to critique the character's feelings and behaviours. For what concerns Brecht, or at least the Brecht of the anti-Aristotelian theatre, acting can either be a form of unconscious re-enactment that perpetuates itself in a sort of contagion from actor to spectator, or a conscious intellectual operation achieved through the power of reason. It must be noted, however, that Brecht's opposition between feeling and reason, if not absolute for what concerns the spectator's experience, as I showed in Chapter 1, will also be relinquished in relation to the actor, when his increasing experience of the stage will convince Brecht that such dichotomy is untenable. Of this, I will write in Chapter 6.

Twentieth-century approaches to acting, such as Brecht's and Stanislavski's, to mention but two of the most renowned, have accustomed us to problematizing the actor's emotional experience in relation to her interpretation of a character, and the epic actor stands for the prototype of the emotionally dis-identified actor. But Brecht was not the originator of this concept. It is in fact in the eighteenth century that the tenet of a 'feeling actor' is for the first time called into question. Although theories of acting can be found across all times, the eighteenth century is of particular interest because, for the first time in history, the actor becomes a privileged object of enquiry, as opposed to the preceding standpoint which considered acting to fall within the sphere of rhetoric (Mazzocut-Mis, 2010). Rhetorical theory, originated in classical texts of ancient Greece and Rome, stipulated that a poetic or dramatic text required an emotional participation on the part of the author in its composition as well as of the orator or actor in its rendition (Vicentini, 2000: 5–6). This is paradigmatically exemplified by Horace's famous passage in the *Ars Poetica* (102–103):[1] 'If you would have me weep, you must first feel grief yourself', which remains a familiar trope in eighteenth-century treatises on the art of the actor as the relic of rhetorical principles.

Within the boundaries of rhetorical theory, the emotional participation of the author and actor to the emotions of the characters is necessarily subservient to the final expressive aim of reaching the spectator so that he will also feel the emotions displayed (Vicentini, 2011). While the tenet of a spectator who shall feel the characters' emotions is hardly challenged in the eighteenth century, it is the function of the actor's feelings which is decisively put into question. In fact the eighteenth century will forever undermine the belief in the doctrine exemplified by Horace's dictum and the text that best testifies to this proposition is the *Paradoxe sur le comédien* by the French philosopher and encyclopaedist Denis Diderot. The *Paradoxe sur le comédien* (hereafter cited as *Paradoxe*) was published posthumously in 1830. The nearly fifty years which elapsed between the death of its author and its first edition symbolize the bridging nature of this work, which projects itself into the future to become a seminal work for nineteenth- and twentieth-century contentions on acting (Vicentini, 2000), but through contemporary references, also roots itself in the theories which developed in the decades preceding its composition, representing the climax of a debate which travels across the eighteenth century and across Europe. In order to analyze in depth the question of the actor's feelings, the *Paradoxe* needs to be read in juxtaposition to its direct and indirect sources, which were unfortunately dismissed and grossly distorted by Diderot, and their misrepresentation perpetuated until the most recent scholarship, as we shall see in the next chapter.

The *Paradoxe* of the actor

The composition of the *Paradoxe* may be dated to the years between 1770 and 1773 (Wilson, 1972: 620) and had been occasioned by the publication, in 1770, of the treatise *Garrick ou les acteurs anglois* (Sticotti, 1770), which Diderot reviewed in an article published in the *Correspondance littéraire*,[2] where he anticipated the contents of his posthumously published essay. The *Paradoxe* is written as a dialogue between two *interlocuteurs*, called *Premier* and *Second*. *Premier*, who is Diderot himself, carries the arguments and counterarguments, while *Second* has the predominant function of being an attentive listener and facilitating the unfolding of Diderot's reasoning through his docile questioning. Famously, the *Paradoxe* proposes that good actors do not feel the emotions of the characters they impersonate, because great actors are deprived of sensibility whereas actors who feel are mediocre at most: 'Extreme sensibility makes middling actors; middling sensibility makes the ruck of bad actors; in complete absence of sensibility is the possibility of a sublime actor' (Diderot, 1883: 17).[3] This is the crux of the *Paradoxe*, that actors must absolutely be deprived of sensibility (*sensibilité*) in order to excel in their profession.

According to Diderot there are two opposite styles of acting, each typified by two famous actresses of his time. Mademoiselle Dumesnil is ruled by sensibility and she 'goes by Nature alone' (Diderot, 1883: 4), whereby *Premier* means that she does not make much effort in learning her part, nor applies her reason to the understanding of it. This supposedly inferior actress instinctively expresses her own spontaneous emotions, in the same manner as the 'man of sensibility obeys the impulse of Nature and gives nothing more or less than the cry of his very heart' (Diderot, 1883: 46). As a consequence, her playing is inconsistent and can only grant success in sporadic moments during a performance: 'She comes on the stage without knowing what she is going to say; half the time she does not known what she is saying: but she has one sublime moment' (Diderot, 1883: 12). Poles apart is the great actress Mademoiselle Clairon, 'who plays from thought, from study of human nature' (Diderot, 1883: 9); she measures, combines, learns, arranges the performance to a degree of precision that can only increase with repetition and will never risk being random or unequal. Clairon is the epitome of the acting style deprived of sensibility: her merit is that she represents the character not through the idiosyncrasies of her own personality, but through the construction of an ideal model (*modèle idéal*) (Diderot, 1883: 9). The talent of the actor lies in her ability to substitute feeling with the 'rendering so exactly the outward signs of feeling' (Diderot, 1883: 16)[4] that spectators will be tricked into believing that she is as emotionally aroused as they are. But in actual fact she has not engaged her emotions, only her bodily exertion. Although *Premier* concedes that she may well be affected by feelings in her first approach to her part during the rehearsal stage, eventually she will reach the point of mastering her role without any emotional involvement because she will play her ideal model from skilful imitation.

Taken as a paradigm for future reflections on acting, Diderot's codification appears to forecast Brecht's opposition between the all-feeling actor of the Aristotelian theatre and the intellectual actor of the epic theatre. Yet there is an important distinction to be made: Diderot's great actor does not aim at inviting the audience into being dispassionate observers of her character; on the contrary, she is paradoxical precisely because she must create the illusion of feeling so that the audience is induced to feel in emotional identification with the character. Paradoxical actors entice spectators into believing that they are partaking of the same emotional experience that overtakes the audience, but it is mere deception because, as *Premier* proclaims, the actor 'feels neither trouble, nor sorrow, nor depression, nor weariness of soul. All these emotions he has given to you. The actor is tired, you are unhappy; he has exertion without feeling, you feeling without exertion' (Diderot, 1883: 16–17).[5]

If the actor's emotional detachment is not aimed at impeding the spectator's emotional identification with the character, the question must be asked of what Diderot supposes to be its purpose. Paradoxically, the actor's lack of sensibility is assumed to enhance the audience's emotional arousal. As *Premier* explains, the stage is governed by conventions, and emotions on the stage are very differently expressed than in real life. Emotions are more spontaneous in relation to real-life events, and their expression makes a very different impression than on a stage: true emotions may well be suited for everyday social intercourse, but 'now transfer your easy tone, your simple expression, your every-day bearing, to the stage, and, I assure you, you will be paltry and weak. You may cry to your heart's content, and the audience will only laugh' (Diderot, 1883: 18–19). Reciprocally, the actor's display of emotions on the stage must appear unnatural in everyday life. *Premier* invites *Second* to imagine Clairon's real expression of feeling in an ordinary situation: 'I must show you Clairon in the real transports of anger. If in them she happened to preserve the bearing, the accent, the action of the stage, with all its artifice and emphasis, [. . .] could you contain your laughter?' (Diderot, 1883: 73). The gap between theatrical and real emotional expression is not only due to theatrical conventions such as the amplitude of the performance space and its relation to the auditorium, or the need for the actor to move from emotion to emotion following the pace of the play's narrative, or the necessity for actors to impersonate different characters in different plays; it is also the fact that fictional characters have a symbolic status well beyond the person of the actor. As *Premier* points out: 'A sure way to act in a cramped, mean style, is to play one's own character. You are, let us say, a tartuffe, a miser, a misanthrope; you may play your part well enough, but you will not come near what the poet has done. He has created *the* Tartuffe, *the* Miser, *the* Misanthrope' (Diderot, 1883: 49), ideal types which typify a social characteristic, like a vice, and not a particular individual.

The crucial concept insisted upon by *Premier* is that sensibility depends on one's own idiosyncratic nature, and this remains in absolute opposition to the ability to understand human nature in its infinite forms: 'sensibility is diametrically opposed to the spirit of the part' because the actor's principal quality 'is the faculty of knowing and imitating all natures' (Diderot, 1883: 55). And Diderot absolutely rejects the idea that sensibility may be associated with this quality. As *Premier* declares:

> It would be a strange abuse of language to give the name of sensibility to this faculty of reproducing all natures, even ferocious natures. Sensibility, according to the only acceptation yet given of the term, is, as it seems to me, that disposition which accompanies organic weakness, which follows on easy affection of the diaphragm, on vivacity of imagination, on delicacy of nerves, which inclines one to being compassionate, to being horrified, to admiration, to fear, to being upset, to tears, to faintings, to rescues, to flights, to exclamations, to loss of self-control, to being contemptuous, disdainful, to having no clear notion of what is true, good, and fine, to being unjust, to going mad.
> (Diderot, 1883: 56)

Whilst this definition of sensibility accords with some prevailing renditions of the eighteenth century, it is very different from the use of sensibility that develops within the writings on the art of the actor which represent the background references of the *Paradoxe*, including the treatise *Garrick ou les acteurs anglois* against which *Premier* sets his argument at the beginning of the dialogue. Diderot's notion of sensibility grounds on an absolute antithesis between sensibility and judgement, which applies not only to actors but extends to humanity at large. Because sensibility ultimately leads to loss of self-control, madness even, if an actor were full of it she would lose her self-possession and the ability to control her performance. That is why, as *Premier* explains, the actor 'must have a deal of judgement. He must have in himself an unmoved and disinterested onlooker. He must have, consequently, penetration and no sensibility' (Diderot, 1883: 7),[6] a definition strikingly evocative of Brecht's (1950) metaphor of the actor as the eyewitness at a street accident.

The dichotomy between sensibility and judgement extends beyond considerations of acting and comes to represent Diderot's (1883: 14) view of society:

> In the great play, the play of the world, the play to which I am constantly recurring, the stage is held by the fiery souls, and the pit is filled with men of genius. The actors are in other words madmen; the spectators, whose business it is to paint their madness, are sages.

In the real world, men and women of feeling lose their self-control to the point of extravagance or even madness, and fall prey to the sober power of observation of talented writers, painters and, indeed, proper actors, who will depict their frenzies in their works of art. While sensibility brings humanity to excessive feeling, men of genius such as great poets, actors, or any other artists, 'being gifted with fine imagination, with broad judgement, with exquisite tact, with a sure touch of taste, are the least sensitive of all creatures' (Diderot, 1883: 13).[7] As Diderot denies that sensibility can ever be a mark of genius, he takes us by surprise when he admits, toward the end of the dialogue, that 'if Nature ever moulded a sensitive soul that soul is mine' (Diderot, 1883: 80) and he describes an episode when he makes himself ridiculous by expressing his sensibility in an enthusiastic and deeply affected response to hearing of the success of one of Sedaine's plays:

> I throw my arms round his neck, my voice fails me, and tears run down my cheeks. There you have the man of sensibility, the middling man. Sedaine, reserved and still, looks at me and says, 'Ah! Monsieur Diderot, you are splendid!' There you have the man of observation – the man of genius.
>
> (Diderot, 1883: 40)

If sensibility is the mark of mediocrity, it does however grant the gift for compassion. Conversely, the ability to simulate feelings which is paradigmatic of the great actor, ultimately leads to an unflattering analogy with hypocrites and deceivers: the actor 'weeps as might weep an unbelieving priest preaching of the Passion; as a seducer might weep at the feet of a woman whom he does not love, but on whom he would impose; like a beggar in the street or at the door of a church – a beggar who substitutes insult for vain appeal; or like a courtesan who has no heart, and who abandons herself in your arms' (Diderot, 1883: 17). The detachment of the actor, guarantee of a perfected and consistent performance, comes to correspond to a cynicism which extends to her private life. Actors, remarks *Premier*, are not easily touched even by their own griefs; off the stage, they are

> polished, caustic, and cold; proud, light of behaviour, spendthrifts, self-interested; struck rather by our absurdities than touched by our misfortunes; masters of themselves at the spectacle of an untoward incident or the recital of a pathetic story; isolated, vagabonds, at the command of the great; little conduct, no friends, scarce any of those holy and tender ties which associate us in the pains and pleasures of another, who in turn shares our own.
>
> (Diderot, 1883: 63)

This moral condemnation of the person of the actor, derives from Diderot's puzzling notion of the role of sensibility: its operations are at the basis of human compassion and fellowship, but also of an incapacity for judgement which can lead to madness; on the other hand, that absence of sensibility which is the foundation of rational insight and even genius, equates to hypocrisy, deception, selfishness. Thus, Diderot's dichotomous classification of actors leads to very different, even opposite, implications to Brecht's, whose epic actor's restraint of feeling is instrumental to her social awareness and political engagement. The contrasting conclusions drawn by Diderot and Brecht from their championing of the unfeeling actor are intriguing to say the least and make it imperative to unravel the conundrum of the actor's sensibility, an enigma which continues to fascinate and remains unresolved.

The *Paradoxe* analyzed

Seemingly evocative of Brecht's polarization of reason and feeling, Diderot's absolute opposition between sensibility and judgement in the art of the actor is based on rather different premises. As we have seen, Brecht accepted feelings as useful to intellectual and social criticism, as long as they were generated by the rational examination of a situation, and he distinguished between feelings generated by empathy and those generated by reason. Diderot instead viewed sensibility and the emotions it engenders as always self-referential. Sensibility disposes actors and, indeed, all human beings to express their own idiosyncratic nature, that is to say, their personal feelings; sensibility is never at the service of understanding the emotional experience of others. This situation is illustrated by Diderot's anecdote of his outburst of emotions on hearing about the success of Sedaine's play. Given that *Premier* openly associates sensibility to compassion and human fellowship, it would seem that sensibility should grant at least at some level an experience of resonance with the feelings of others. And yet, Sedaine's sardonic comment 'Ah! Monsieur Diderot, you are splendid' (Diderot, 1883: 40) shows that Diderot's supposedly sympathetic response to Sedaine is utterly misplaced.

The philosopher's view of sensibility should be understood within the development that the concept underwent in the second half of the eighteenth century. Sensibility, which has been described as a 'period marker' of the eighteenth century (Csengei, 2011: 5), became pertinent to several different disciplines, from philosophy and ethics, to medicine and physiology, aesthetics and literature (Vila, 1998: 1). This proliferation of meanings is particularly relevant to Diderot's rendition, considering that the editing of the *Encyclopédie* and his eclectic interests exposed him to the most updated knowledge on the subject. Within the abundance of different definitions that the word enjoyed, sensibility stood for the means through which human beings could access their 'natural goodness, benevolence and compassion' (Csengei, 2011: 5). However, it also carried an intrinsic ambivalence, implying 'a potential dangerous quality that could lead to emotional excess, moral degeneracy, and physical debilitation' (Vila, 1998: 1). *Premier* points to this aspect of sensibility when it defines it as the propensity not only to compassion and vivacity of imagination, but also to loss of self-control, injustice, extravagance and even madness (Diderot, 1883: 56). In the *Paradoxe*, Diderot's statements about sensibility carry an inconsistency compatible with that found in his contemporary cultural milieu. On the one hand, sensibility has a positive connotation as the quality which supports bonding between human beings, and lack of it is the precondition for a selfish and deceitful personality. On the other hand, sensibility is a hindrance to rationality and an absolute contraindication to genius.

The sheer opposition between sensibility and judgement is somewhat surprising in Diderot, given that the philosopher had previously expressed views aligned to the philosophical principles of sensism. Developed in France mainly by Condillac on the basis of Locke's theories, sensism postulated that all knowledge and all psychic operations, including reflection and reason, derive from sensation and affect (Cassirer, 1951). In his *Philosophical Thoughts*, an early work of 1746, Diderot fully endorses the notion that reason is founded on feelings. Paraphrasing the philosopher's words, Cassirer (1951: 107–108) explains that according to Diderot:

> It is of no avail to oppose the passions, and it would be the height of the ridiculous to try to destroy them since in so doing we should undermine the proud foundations of reason. Everything excellent in poetry, painting, and music, everything sublime in art and morals, is derived from this source. Hence the affects must not be weakened but strengthened; for the true power of the soul springs from the harmonious balance of the passions.

Here, Diderot's view is clearly at odds with the one he expresses in the *Paradoxe*, and it highlights that his opinion of the status of emotions in relation to reason will vary at different points of his intellectual work. In fact, the examination of Diderot's reflections on acting prior to the *Paradoxe* reveals an equivalent inconsistency and oscillation in his appraisal of the function of emotions, as I shall discuss later in the chapter.

The notion that sensations and feelings are at the basis of all mental activities is extended by some eighteenth-century philosophers to considerations about morality. It is in this context that sensibility comes to be associated with compassion and sympathy. However, as it was for sensibility, eighteenth-century definitions of sympathy are also disparate and inconsistent (Csengei, 2011: 31). According to Hume, for instance, sympathy is based on:

> an interpersonal transmission and communication of emotions. In Book 2 ('Of the Passions') of the *Treatise of Human Nature* (1739–40), he writes that we can feel what another person feels, because we 'receive by communication their inclinations and sentiments, however different from, or even contrary to our own'.
>
> (Csengei, 2011: 40–41)

It follows that sensibility should warrant that sympathy is truly grounded in experiencing the emotions of the person we feel for. But this is not what Diderot seems to imply when he relates of his encounter with Sedaine. The incongruous nature of his and Sadaine's feelings seems rather to tally with Adam Smith's notion of the sympathetic imagination. Despite developing his moral philosophy on the basis of

Hume's proposition that emotions are the foundations of morality, in his *Theory of Moral Sentiments*, first published in 1759, Smith denies Hume's assertion that emotions are directly communicated from person to person. In the opening paragraphs of his treatise, he writes:

> As we have no immediate experience of what other men feel, we can form no idea of the manner in which they are affected, but by conceiving what we ourselves should feel in the like situation. Though our brother is upon the rack, as long as we ourselves are at our ease, our senses will never inform us of what he suffers. They never did, and never can, carry us beyond our own person, and it is by the imagination only that we can form any conception of what are his sensations. Neither can that faculty help us to this any other way, than by representing to us what would be our own, if we were in his case.
>
> (Smith, 1976: 9)

As has been rightly pointed out, this premise leads to characterizing sympathy as a fundamentally solipsistic enterprise (Csengei, 2011: 32). The bearer of sympathy cannot know what the other person feels through direct communication of the sufferer's experience, and must therefore rely on her imagination about how she would feel in a comparable situation. Accordingly, Diderot's feelings for Sedaine are the product of imagining how he – Diderot – would have felt if one of his own plays had been as successful as Sedaine's. The construction of sympathy on self-centred feelings fully corresponds to a view of sensibility as entirely self-referential.

The *Paradoxe* of the actor stands on the conjunction of two propositions concerning sensibility: that sensibility is incompatible with judgement and reason, and that sensibility is about one's own personal feelings. This naturally leads to the presumption that either people are engrossed in sensibility, in which case they feel and express their own emotions within a solipsistic experience, or they are deprived of sensibility, and can therefore engage reason and judgement in order to understand the emotions of others, but from a purely intellectual and detached stance. The art of the actor, as we have seen, exemplifies this schism.

About David Garrick

In the *Paradoxe*, Diderot invokes the example of the great actor David Garrick, with whom he was personally acquainted, to support his theory of the unfeeling actor. In some way this was a necessary ploy, given that Garrick had been presented by Sticotti as the paradigmatic example of the feeling actor, as the title of his book, *Garrick ou les acteurs anglois*, testifies. Diderot recalls having seen Garrick place his head between two doors and show in quick succession a sequence of very different emotional expressions:

> from wild delight to temperate pleasure, from this to tranquillity, from tranquillity to surprise, from surprise to blank astonishment, from that to sorrow, from sorrow to the air of one overwhelmed, from that to fright, from fright

> to horror, from horror to despair, and thence he will go up again to the point from which he started.
>
> (Diderot, 1883: 38)

This extremely skilful performance convinces the philosopher of the impossibility that the English actor may have reached his masterly effect through feeling, proving that Garrick's greatness was indeed based on detached observation and deft imitation. There is however a difficulty: Diderot has to contend with Garrick's own admission to feeling deeply when he acts. To overcome his predicament, the philosopher applies his definition of sensibility to the interpretation of Garrick's account of his acting practice:

> I take thee to witness, Roscius of England, celebrated Garrick; thee, who by the unanimous consent of all existing nations art held for the greatest actor they have known! Now render homage to truth. Hast thou not told me that, despite thy depth of feeling, thy action would be weak if, whatever passion or character thou hadst to render, thou couldst not raise thyself by the power of thought to the grandeur of a Homeric shape with which though soughtest to identify thyself? When I replied that it was not then from thine own type thou didst play, confess thine answer. Didst not avow avoiding this with care, and say that thy playing was astounding only because thou didst constantly exhibit a creature of the imagination which was not thyself?
>
> (Diderot, 1883: 60)[8]

Garrick's admission that he plays an imagined character, what Diderot (1883: 9) calls an 'ideal model', is enough for denying Garrick the status of a feeling actor, as this latter would amount to Garrick playing himself. Perhaps not wanting to go as far as suggesting that a great actor like Garrick is utterly deceived in his knowledge of his art, Diderot (1883: 95)[9] comments that 'to have sensibility is one thing, to feel [*sentir*] is another. One is a matter of soul, the other of judgement'. Willing to do anything in order to support his argument, he adds to that vagueness and ambiguity of the language used to describe acting that he himself seems to deplore at the outset of the *Paradoxe* (Diderot, 1883: 6). It should also be noted, for the sake of completeness, that elsewhere in the *Paradoxe*, *Premier* had suggested that actors are well aware of their lack of feeling but they guard it as their secret (Diderot, 1883: 15). Diderot's incitation to Garrick to 'confess' may subtly imply that actors do not like to make certain technical tools of their profession known to the public.

Nevertheless, if Garrick had ever known the *Paradoxe*, he would most likely have disapproved of it. A passage from Garrick's correspondence not only shows him to abide by the idea of the feeling actor, but also reveals his disapproval of Madame Clairon, precisely on that quality of detachment and control which Diderot so much praises. In a letter of 1769 he wrote:

> [Clairon] has everything that art and a good understanding, with great natural spirit, can give her. But then I fear [. . .] the heart has none of those

> instantaneous feelings, that life-blood, that keen sensibility, that bursts at once from genius, and, like electrical fire, shoots through the veins, marrow, bones and all, of every spectator. Madame *Clairon* is so conscious and certain of what she can do, that she never, I believe, had the feelings of the instant come upon her unexpectedly: but I pronounce that the greatest strokes of genius have been unknown to the actor himself, till circumstances, and the warmth of the scene has sprung the mine as it were, as much to his own surprise, as that of the audience. Thus I make a great difference between a great genius and a good actor. The first will always realize the feelings of his character, and be transported beyond himself [. . .].
>
> (Garrick, 1831: 359)

Diderot's supposition that Garrick and Clairon shared the same acting practice would have hardly flattered the English actor. This however remains speculation given that, of course, Garrick could have never responded to the *Paradoxe*.

Dual consciousness and the psychology of acting

It was in 1888, fifty years following the publication of the *Paradoxe*, but more than a hundred after its composition, that another Englishman took it upon himself to disprove Diderot's theory by directly consulting the opinion of great actors: William Archer, a drama critic and writer, put Diderot's theory to a sort of experimental test. His preoccupation with the *Paradoxe* had brought him to question the validity of a theory that sprang out of a dialogue between 'a dogmatic First and a docile Second', rather than, as he would have wished, between 'a trained psychologist and an experienced and versatile actor' (Archer, 1888: 3). In Archer's view, Diderot's dialogue was the rambling speech of a philosopher who, dissatisfied with his own theory, was not prepared to admit it and rather imposed his ideas on the reader as *Premier* forces them on the 'dumb' *Second*. Archer's appraisal of Diderot's work is clearly limiting given the enormous influence that the book has had on future scholarship, 'by establishing itself as the paradigmatic text in its field' (Roach, 1993: 117). However it is in turn consequential at least for two reasons: first, it reveals and dismantles some of the key errors in Diderot's argument; secondly, it calls on the authority of actors to address the conundrum of their art in a systematic way.

That Diderot used some of the terminology in a problematic way, as I pointed out earlier, is a strong objection of Archer's. In particular it is the use of the term 'sensibility' ['*sensibilité*'] that disturbs him. If sensibility is what Diderot assumes it to be, 'Hysteria, surely, is a much apter name for the disease' (Archer, 1888: 36). Incidentally, it needs to be clarified that Diderot's understanding of '*sensibilité*' as excessive and misplaced feeling did not have a connotation of femininity as the term 'hysteria' used by Archer seems to imply. As has been shown,

> French writers did not polarize sensibility in relation to sex and gender nearly as much as did their British counterparts, at least not until the last few

> decades of the century; rather, even the most hard-boiled philosophes prided themselves on their sensibility and saw nothing unmanly about cultivating this quality.
>
> (Vila, 1998: 3)

For Archer, the main difficulty with Diderot's rendition of sensibility is his forced assumption that the only alternative to the ideally unfeeling and expressive actor is an actor so engrossed in feelings (or rather hysteria) that her power of expression gets overthrown. As Archer (1888: 89) points out:

> the use of inward emotion is to reinforce, not to supplant, outward expression. No one has ever doubted that the actor must be able to express what he feels, or feeling will avail him to nothing. The question at issue is whether he ought, or ought not, to feel what he expresses.

To avoid these errors and more, Archer wished, as I mentioned, for a constructive dialogue between a psychologist and a distinguished actor. Despite being no psychologist, he believed that by interrogating actors he could at least avoid that mistake, which Diderot makes all too often, of making false assumptions about actors' methods, as the example of Garrick proves. By questioning as many prominent actors as he could reach with a written questionnaire, he hoped to arrive at more reliable conclusions than Diderot's. Through his systematic collection of responses, Archer establishes that great actors (or indeed the majority of them) do actually feel while they act and that they consider this 'feeling' status to be their most powerful means of communicating with the audience. In order to invalidate the objection that actors may think they feel or perhaps may like to mislead others into thinking it, while they actually don't, Archer asks actors to report about physical signs of emotions during their performances. He believes that signs like shedding tears, speaking in a broken voice, or, even more, blushing or paling, cannot be feigned; their abundant presence, testified by lots of his respondents, proves beyond question that actors in performance are truly feeling.

Having established that the actor feels, Archer (1888: 195) asks a second crucial question: whether she ought to feel. The importance of this point lies, in essence, with what Archer identifies as the problem of expression: actors ought to feel if by doing so they enhance their expressive capabilities and ultimately their effect on the spectators. His respondents are vastly in favour of this notion, providing Archer with a solid argument to dismantle Diderot's paradox of an actor who does not feel in order to make a spectator feel. Such operation re-establishes order into a theory which goes back to ancient rhetoric and has been universally adhered to, including by Shakespeare, as Archer (1888: 44) is eager to point out. But dismantling a paradox may sometimes have the effect of generating a different one, and such is the case here. Archer does not wish to object to Diderot's illustrations, of which there are several in the *Paradoxe*, of the actor's ability to control her performance with a degree of shrewdness. For instance, *Premier* describes the instance when during an intensively dramatic moment of a performance, an actress, piqued by the burst of laughter in the audience, turns to harangue them:

> Duclos, who was playing Inez, was angered, and cried to the pit: 'Laugh, you blockheads, at the finest point in the piece!' The pit listened, and was silent; the actress went on with her part, and her tears and the spectators' flowed together.
>
> (Diderot, 1883: 46)

Examples such as this pose the dilemma whether a state of awareness of one's surroundings is compatible with the actor feeling her character's emotions. Archer puts this question to his respondents and collects a series of illustrations about situations in which they were acting in full emotional identification with the character while also able to respond to situations extraneous to the character's actions or feelings, but rather concerning them as a person. One case in point is an incident reported by the great Italian actor Salvini, who once found himself in the embarrassing situation of feeling the belt of his trousers giving away during a passionate scene: artfully, 'he dashed at a tiger-skin which covered the divan and swathed it round his body [. . .] "I was told," he says, "that I had never played the scene with greater intensity of rage, irony and despair" ' (Archer, 1888: 163).

Supplying plenty of similar examples, Archer demonstrates that actors declare that while they engage in activities which are simultaneous but extraneous to the performance, they also continue to feel the character's emotions. To prove this point with the testimony of real actors was particularly relevant to a dismantling of the *Paradoxe*'s argument, because Diderot had used a number of examples of actors' ability to step out of character during a performance as a proof that they do not feel. One of his most conspicuous anecdotes had been of a married couple who, while playing two lovers in one of Molière's plays, engaged in a simultaneous bickering, conducting the two dialogues, the theatrical and the real-life one, simultaneously, without the audience ever realizing (Diderot, 1883: 32–34). Indeed, as *Premier* claims, artistically 'they surpassed themselves [. . .] they excited continual bursts of applause from pit and boxes; a scene interrupted half-a-score of times with our clapping of hands and exclamations of delight' (Diderot, 1883: 32). If for Diderot this dialogue conducted on a double plane was the proof that the actors were not feeling, Archer contests that such proof is invalid, because there is a better explanation than lack of feeling for the ability of the actors to carry out their double dialogue simultaneously.

Having brought the authority of the best actors of his time to support his repudiation of the *Paradoxe*'s contentions, Archer (1888: 150)[10] puts forth an alternative and much preferred explanation for the question of feeling in the actor's art: 'The real paradox of acting, it seems to me, resolves itself into the paradox of dual consciousness'. What does Archer intend by dual consciousness? That actors' brains can engage in a double or multiple action: they can feel the character's emotions while also being aware of their surroundings and conscious that they are a different person from the character. Incidentally, a very similar notion had been offered by James Boswell (1929) in his essay *On the profession of a player* published in *The London Magazine* in 1770, the same year that saw in France the appearance of the treatise *Garrick ou les acteurs anglois* by Sticotti. Boswell (1929: 13), like Sticotti, took Garrick's practice as the quintessence of great acting and correctly supposed that the English actor would declare to be feeling while performing:

> I am persuaded that Mr. Garrick will tell us, that it is easy to him to play a part in which the passions display themselves naturally. In such a part, when he is once entered into the character, its different effusions are like the effusions of his own mind.

But Boswell (1929: 14–15) was also troubled by the idea of considering the emotional identification of an actor with her character as an absolute state of mind:

> I am aware that my proposition, that a player is really and truly the character in which he appears, may be misrepresented; and I remember to have heard the most illustrious author of this age, whose conversation is thought by many even to excel his writings, exert his eloquence against this proposition, and with the luxuriance of humour for which he is distinguished, render it exceedingly ridiculous: 'If, sir,' said he, 'Garrick believes himself to be every character that he represents, he is a madman and ought to be confined. Nay, sir, he is a villain, and ought to be hanged. [. . .] If, sir, he has really been that person in his own mind, he has in his own mind been as guilty as Macbeth'.

As it was for Diderot, there is a suspicion or derision – here expressed by the 'illustrious author' Samuel Johnson, whom Boswell takes as his authority – of the idea that actors play themselves, that their emotional identification with a character ultimately amounts to believing in being the character. Boswell's (1929: 17–18) response to the absurdity of an actor who has fallen mad, or in modern terms, suffers from a psychotic illness, is the concept of 'double feeling':

> If I may be allowed to conjecture what is the nature of that mysterious power by which a player really is the character which he represents, my notion is, that he must have a kind of double feeling. He must assume in a strong degree the character which he represents, while he at the same time retains the consciousness of his own character. The feelings and passions of the character which he represents must take full possession as it were of the antechamber of his mind, while his own character remains in the innermost recess.

The concept of double feeling is very close to William Archer's idea of dual consciousness and possibly its precursor. It has even been suggested (Roach, 1993: 147–148) that it is first expressed in the *Paradoxe* itself, when *Premier*, talking about Clairon performing dispassionately but extremely skilfully her ideal model, 'has a double personality; that of the little Clairon and of the great Agrippina' (Diderot, 1883: 11).

It is of note that Boswell specifies that double feeling pertains to all human beings, not just the actor. As he puts it: 'The double feeling which I have mentioned is experienced by many men in the common intercourse of life. Were nothing but the real character to appear, society would not be half so safe and agreeable as we find it' (Boswell, 1929: 19). Archer's (1888: 151) declaration as to the universality of dual consciousness is even more unequivocal:

> I looked upon the double action of the brain as a matter of universal experience, a thing to be assumed just as one assumes that the normal man has two legs. I did not regard it as a tendency peculiar to actors, but common to all men.

Their formulation of double feeling or dual consciousness turns out to be a universal truth concerning the human mind, raising the question of whether it is legitimate to invoke it as the core of the actor's art. Archer (1888: 150) himself admits it to be in itself a paradox. As has been pointed out, 'Diderot splits the actor into two to free the actor from having to feel at the moment of performance. Archer splits the actor in two to make feeling possible' (Mazer, 2015: 27). In point of fact, it is disquieting that dual consciousness advances a psychological explanation that is not that different from the one proposed in the *Paradoxe*: actors are deemed to be champions in dissociating their feelings from their consciousness, whether they do it to obliterate them completely or to let them flow without disturbing the rational mind.

Diderot's ideas on acting preceding the Paradoxe

Diderot's initial engagement with theatrical matters precedes the writing of the *Paradoxe* by about fifteen years and lies in his attempts to establish a new form of drama, which he calls *le genre sérieux*, as opposed to the classical taxonomical genres of comedy and tragedy. His project is that of a playwright and of a theorist. In 1757 he writes his first play, *Le Fils naturel*, followed the next year by *Le Père de famille.* Each play is accompanied by a significant exposition of theory, respectively in *Les Entretiens sur Le Fils naturel*, a triplet of dialogues supposedly between Diderot and Dorval, author of the play, and in *De la poésie dramatique*, a more conventional treatise on theatrical matters addressed to his friend Grimm. Because the discourse of these works is somewhat dominated by dramaturgy, the preoccupation with acting is fairly marginal. Nevertheless, it is significant.

Like the *Paradoxe*, the *Entretiens sur Le Fils naturel* (hereafter cited as *Entretiens*) are structured as a dialogue between Diderot and Dorval, the supposed author of the play *Le Fils naturel*. Allegedly, Dorval is an amateur playwright eager to promote a form of playwriting centred on '*vraisemblance*': his quest for truthfulness extends to all aspects of dramatic composition, such as thematic choices, which need to reflect real and realistic facts, or the dramatization, which should favour the Aristotelian unities in as much as they are at the service, not the disservice, of realism (Diderot, 1939: 85–89). Following a domino effect, '*vraisemblance*' becomes a concern in relation to acting; and what could be more apt to study the scope of this subject than Dorval's project, to put actors in the condition to play themselves? The ploy of *Le Fils naturel* is that Dorval has based the play entirely on a true fact which has occurred to him and his family and that he has called the life-protagonists of the event to become protagonists on stage of the dramatization of the event itself. The *Entretiens* represent Dorval/Diderot's experimentation with the absolute correspondence between fiction and reality, both on the plane of dramatic writing and on that of acting. But in actual fact they are an utterly fictional game. The play, supposedly a dramatization of a real event (Diderot, 1939: 19–21), is rather the adaptation of a subplot of the Italian comedy *Il vero amico* by Goldoni (1939), first published in 1751 (Mittman, 1973). The actors are supposed to be people made of flesh and blood, who have lived through the events described in the play as well as performed them, while their reality is twice removed because their existence is constructed through the sparse references of the *Entretiens* (Hobson, 1974). The dialogues of the *Entretiens* are allegedly the transcription of Diderot's conversations with Dorval, Diderot even scrupling to point out that such transcription may not do justice to Dorval's impromptu words. In actual fact, Dorval is Diderot's alter ego and the spokesman for Diderot's own ideas and the dialogues express Diderot's musings.

Notwithstanding being a philosophical rather than a real experiment with actors, the *Entretiens* present Diderot's beliefs about acting during his first activity as playwright. Interestingly, this experiment is grounded on the proposition of an absolute coincidence between the character and the person of the actor, and on the conviction that it is possible to transpose the expression of emotions from the '*salon*' (literally, the living room) to the stage. Dorval advocates that acting should be based on a realistic performance, where tone of voice, gesture and stage movements are as close as possible to those of domestic life, and he requests that his play be judged according to the standards of domestic truth (Diderot, 1939: 92–95). Dorval also observes that during the rehearsals of the play, his fellow actors, namely his family relations, were influenced in their performance by their present feelings, even if asked to act according to the emotions they experienced during the actual event of which the play is a dramatization. He gives the example of how the increased tenderness between the spouses (himself and Constance, and Clairville and Rosalie) led them to perform the harsher events depicted in the play with softer tones. The fact that the actors' personal feelings impact significantly on the interpretation of the characters (who are nothing more than their previous selves, anyhow) is not of concern to Dorval. Ultimately, this is consistent with his championing of sensibility in the art of the actor. As he maintains, an actress of mediocre intelligence but great sensibility can reach the heights of emotional expression: she finds the right expression for the feelings she needs to represent without having to give it conscious thought (Diderot, 1939: 108); she acts, one could say paraphrasing Dorval, as if by instinct. Dorval's praise of sensibility extends to value it as the quintessence of all arts; in point of fact he explicitly affirms: 'Poets, actors, musicians, painters, first class singers, great dancers, tender lovers, true devotees, all this enthusiastic and passionate troop feels vividly and reflects little' (Diderot, 1939: 108).[11] Nothing could be more at variance with *Premier*'s statements.

There is a colossal difference between Diderot/Dorval's imaginary experiment on acting in which the coincidence between actor and character is taken to represent the ideal condition of a reformed stage practice, and Diderot/*Premier*'s later formulation of the absolute dissociation between actor's and character's feelings which leads to the extremes of a paradox. At this early stage, Diderot believes that sensibility is the true quality of great actors, and of all talented artists; he decidedly downplays the role of reflection and intelligence; he approves of acting by instinct; and he champions a form of acting in which actors draw on the coincidence between their personal feelings and even their personal life experiences and those of the characters they play. He equates sensibility with the expression of personal feelings and playing one's own nature, in continuity with his later views; he also anticipates the notion that an opposition between sensibility and judgement characterizes acting and all artistic disciplines, although here in favour of sensibility. All these points create a strong, if uncomfortable, impression that the *Paradoxe*'s arguments work extremely well as a confutation, by Diderot, of his own earlier theories. Diderot, however, does not seem, at least in this instance, to be a good judge of his own faults and merits.

Shortly after the publication of his essay *De la poésie dramatique*, Diderot received a letter which was to become notorious, by the actress and later novelist Madame Riccoboni (Marie-Jeanne Laboras de Mezières), whom Diderot mistakenly believed to be a Riccoboni by birth (Courville, 1958: 43, footnote 63). Instead she was the wife of the very François Riccoboni, whose essay on the art of the actor Diderot took to be an anticipation of his theory of the paradoxical actor, as we shall see in the next chapter. The letter (in Diderot, 1994: 121–143) was an attempt by the actress to correct what she perceived to be Diderot's mistaken assumptions on acting due to his lack of specific knowledge of the craft. Diderot, she claimed, did not have first-hand experience of the stage and hence could not understand the rationale behind some of the acting devices that he criticized or wanted to modify. In particular, she was sceptical of the emphasis he put on following the rules of nature: 'The stage can never become as simple as the [living] room; and in order to be truthful at the theatre, one needs to go a little beyond the natural' (in Diderot, 1994: 126).[12] Neither in his response letter to Madame Riccoboni, nor in later writings, will Diderot admit heeding Madame Riccoboni's advice, and in the *Paradoxe* he will actually take the opportunity to name her, on account of her excessive sensibility, and perhaps maliciously, as 'one of the worst actresses that ever appeared on the stage', notably adding that 'No one talks better on dramatic art; no one plays worse' (Diderot, 1883: 85). This same tendency to oversimplify the opinions of others, and to exploit his misrepresentation in order to strengthen his own argument, applies to Diderot's reading of the formulations of acting advanced by the texts that he references in the *Paradoxe*. It is unfortunate that the philosopher's declarations that the *Paradoxe* is a negation of the ideas presented in the book *Garrick ou les acteurs anglois*, have been taken at face value. This has led to the hasty assumption that the theory exposed in this and other related texts is what *Premier* claims it to be. The ensuing misapprehension has engendered a disregard for such theory and a gross misconception of its significance for understanding the role of emotions in the actor's art, as I will show in the next chapter.

Notes

1 'Si vis me flere, dolendum est primum ipsi tibi'. All quotations from Horace's *Ars Poetica* are from: Horace, 'Ars Poetica or Epistle to the Pisos', in *Satires, Epistles and Ars Poetica*, translated by H. R. Fairclough (London: William Heinemann, 1970), pp. 442–489.
2 In: Correspondance littéraire, philosophique et critique de Grimm et de Diderot, depuis 1753 jusqu'en 1790. Nouvelle édition. Tome septième, 1770–1772, pp. 73–84 + pp. 94–105, Paris: Furne et Ladrange (1829).
3 'C'est l'extrême sensibilité qui fait les acteurs médiocres; c'est la sensibilité médiocre qui fait la multitude des mauvais acteurs; et c'est le manque absolu de sensibilité qui prépare les acteurs sublimes' (Diderot, 1994: 46).
4 'rendre si scrupuleusement les signes extérieurs du sentiment' (Diderot, 1994: 45).
5 'il ne lui reste ni trouble, ni douleur, ni mélancolie, ni affaissement d'âme. C'est vous qui remportez toutes ces impressions. L'acteur est las, et vous triste; c'est qu'il s'est démené sans rien sentir, e que vous avez senti sans vous démener' (Diderot, 1994: 46).
6 'je lui veux beaucoup de jugement; il me faut dans cet homme un spectateur froid et tranquille; j'en exige, par conséquent, de la pénétration et nulle sensibilité' (Diderot, 1994: 39).
7 'Les hommes chauds, violents, sensibles, sont en scène; ils donnent le spectacle, mais ils n'en jouissent pas. C'est d'après eux que l'homme de génie fait sa copie. Les grands poètes, les grands acteurs, et peut-être en général tous les grands imitateurs de la nature, quels qu'ils soient, doués d'une belle imagination, d'un grand jugement, d'un tact fin, d'un goût très sûr, sont les êtres les moins sensibles' (Diderot, 1994: 43).
8 'Je te prends à témoin, Roscius anglais, célèbre Garrick [. . .] Ne m'as-tu pas dit que, quoique tu sentisses fortement, ton action serait faible, si, quelle que fût la passion ou le caractère que tu avais à rendre, tu ne savais t'élever par la pensée à la grandeur d'un fantôme homérique auquel tu cherchais à t'identifier? Lorsque je t'objectai que ce n'était donc pas d'après toi que tu jouais, confesse ta réponse: ne m'avouas-tu pas que tu t'en gardais bien, et que tu ne paraissais si étonnant sur la scène, que parce que tu montrais sans cesse au spectacle un être d'imagination qui n'était pas toi?' (Diderot, 1994: 81).
9 'C'est qu'être sensible est une chose, et sentir est une autre. L'une est une affaire d'âme, l'autre une affaire de jugement' (Diderot, 1994: 109).
10 Double consciousness was a word coined in 1880 by the nineteenth-century philosopher and literary critic George Henry Lewes to express an idea already prevalent in discussions of acting of his time (Mazer, 2015: 26). It is also employed by Henry Irving in 1883, in his *Preface* to the first English translation of the *Paradoxe* (Diderot, 1883: xv).
11 'Les poëtes, les acteurs, les musiciens, les peintres, les chanteurs de premier ordre, les grands danseurs, les amants tendres, les vrais dévots, toute cette troupe enthousiaste et passionnée sent vivement, et réfléchit peu'.
12 'La scène ne peut jamais devenir aussi simple que la chambre; et pour être vrai au théâtre, il faut passer un peu le naturel'.

Bibliography

Archer, W. (1888) *Masks or Faces: A Study in the Psychology of Acting*, London: Longmans, Green and Company.
Boswell, J. (1929) *On the Profession of a Player*, London: Elkin Mathews & Marrot.

Brecht, B. (1950) 'The Street Scene: A Basic Model for an Epic Theatre', in *Brecht on Theatre: The Development of an Aesthetic*, edited and translated by J. Willett (2001), London: Methuen, pp. 121–128.
Cassirer, E. (1951) *The Philosophy of the Enlightenment*, Princeton: Princeton University Press.
Courville, X. de (1958) *Luigi Riccoboni dit Lélio. III (1716–1731). La leçon*, Paris: Libraire E. Droz.
Csengei, I. (2011) *Sympathy, Sensibility and the Literature of Feeling in the Eighteenth Century*, Basingstoke: Palgrave Macmillan.
Diderot, D. (1883) *The Paradox of Acting*, translation and annotations by Walter Herries Pollock, London: Chatto & Windus.
Diderot, D. (1939) *Théâtre: Le Fils naturel, Le Joueur, Le Père de famille, De la poésie dramatique*, éditeur J. Assézat, Paris: Libraire Garnier Frères.
Diderot, D. (1994) *Paradoxe sur le comédien. Suivi de Lettres sur le théâtre à Madame Riccoboni et à Mademoiselle Jodin*, éditeur R. Abirached, Paris: Gallimard.
Garrick, D. (1831) *The Private Correspondence of David Garrick with the Most Celebrated Persons of His Time*, now first published from the originals, and illustrated with notes, vol. 1, London: Henry Colburn and Richard Bentley.
Goldoni, C. (1939) 'Il vero amico', in *Tutte le opere di Carlo Goldoni*, a cura di G. Ortolani, Milano: Arnoldo Mondadori Editore, vol. 3, pp. 567–640.
Hobson, M. (1974) 'Notes pour les "Entretiens" sur "Le fils naturel"', *Revue d'histoire littéraire de la France*, 74e Année, vol. 2, pp. 203–213.
Horace (1970) 'Ars Poetica or Epistle to the Pisos', in *Satires, Epistles and Ars Poetica*, translated by H. Rushton Fairclough, London: William Heinemann, pp. 442–489.
Mazer, C.M. (2015) *Double Shakespeares: Emotionalist-Realist Acting and Contemporary Performance*, Madison/Teaneck: Fairleigh Dickinson University Press.
Mazzocut-Mis, M. (2010) 'Presentazione', in *Paradossi settecenteschi. La figura dell'attore nel secolo dei lumi*, edited by M. Accornero, K. Angioletti, M. Bertolini, C. Guaita and E. Oggionni, Milano: Edizioni Universitarie di Lettere, Economia e Diritto, pp. 9–11.
Mittman, B. (1973) 'Diderot's First "Entretien" and Goldoni', *The Modern Language Review*, vol. 68, no. 2, pp. 309–314.
Roach, J.R. (1993) *The Player's Passion: Studies in the Science of Acting*, Ann Arbor: The University of Michigan Press.
Smith, A. (1976) *The Theory of Moral Sentiments*, Oxford: Oxford University Press.
Sticotti, M. (1770) *Garrick ou les Acteurs Anglois. Ouvrage contenant des Observations sur l'Art dramatique, sur l'Art de la Représentation, et le Jeu des Acteurs. Avec des Notes historiques et critiques, et des Anecdotes sur les différents Théâtres de Londres et de Paris*, traduit de l'anglois, seconde édition, augmentée, Paris: J.-P. Costard.
Vicentini, C. (2000) 'Teorie della recitazione. Diderot e la questione del Paradosso', in *Storia del teatro moderno e contemporaneo. Il grande teatro borghese Settecento-Ottocento*, Torino: Einaudi, vol. 2, pp. 5–47.
Vicentini, C. (2011) 'Theory of Acting V: The Birth of Emotionalism', *Acting Archives Essays: Acting Archives Review*, Supplement 5, [Online], Available: http://www.actingarchives.it
Vila, A.C. (1998) *Enlightenment and Pathology: Sensibility in the Literature and Medicine of Eighteenth-Century France*, Baltimore/London: The John Hopkins University Press.
von Held, P. (2011) *Alienation and Theatricality: Diderot after Brecht*, Oxford: Legenda.
Wilson, A.M. (1972) *Diderot*, New York: Oxford University Press.

Chapter 4

The emotionalist theory of acting

Introduction

In the *Paradoxe*, Diderot presents his view on acting as sharply opposed to that exposed in the book against which he takes issue: *Garrick ou les acteurs anglois* (hereafter cited as *Garrick*) by Michel Sticotti. While *Premier* champions judgement and lack of sensibility as the basis of great acting, the author of the *Garrick* has foolishly pleaded the cause of sensibility. This neat contrast, which was later defined by William Archer (1888: 11) in his study on the psychology of acting as the dispute between the emotionalist and anti-emotionalist positions, constitutes the backbone of the *Paradoxe*'s contentions. And yet, looking closely into the *Garrick* and its sources reveals the extent of Diderot's mistaken assumptions and grants a more subtle and truthful rendition of the so-called emotionalist position. As a parallel to his dispute against the *Garrick*, *Premier* makes reference to two other eighteenth-century essays on the art of the actor: 'the question I am diving into was once before started between a middling man of letters, Rémond de Sainte-Albine, and a great actor, Riccoboni. The man of letters pleaded the cause of sensibility; the actor took up my case' (Diderot, 1883: 83). Here Diderot refers respectively to *Le Comédien* by Rémond de Sainte-Albine, first published in 1747, and to *L'Art du théâtre* by François Riccoboni, published in 1750. François Riccoboni's book is called upon to testify of the correctness of *Premier*'s theory, while *Le Comédien* is confined to representing, alongside the *Garrick*, the fallacious argument that *Premier* sets out to refute.

The *Paradoxe* is undoubtedly a paradigmatic text in the history of acting theories, but regrettably, it is rarely examined in relation to its references, namely those texts that *Premier* himself alludes to as pertaining to his discussion. Approaching the *Paradoxe* as a stand-alone system of ideas is partly justified by the much greater fortune that it enjoyed, in circulation and translation, compared to its references, surely a sign of the merit of the work in extending its conceptual reach far beyond questions of acting (Harriman-Smith, 2015: 83). Nevertheless, the notion that with the *Paradoxe* 'Diderot brought much that was new to thinking about performance' (Harriman-Smith, 2015: 85) is misleading. *Premier* indeed mentions 'a great actor' Riccoboni, who, like him, endorsed a view of acting entailing lack of feeling and thus substantiating his argument. Incidentally, in a note to his article in the *Correspondance littéraire*[1] – a first draft, as we shall remember, of the *Paradoxe* – Diderot proves to be misinformed about the Riccoboni family, given that he believes the champion of the unfeeling actor to be the same Riccoboni who authored *La Reformation du théâtre*, whilst the first, François Riccoboni, is actually the son of the second, Luigi Riccoboni. In Chapter 3, I have pointed to a similar instance of mistaken identity with regards to Madame Riccoboni, whom Diderot believed to be a Riccoboni by birth while she was instead François's wife. The Riccobonis, prominent actors at the Italian theatre in Paris, were granted a fairly casual and often inaccurate referencing; a similar fate haunts the Sticottis to this day (Meldolesi, 1969: 29). But on this family issue I will return briefly later.

L'Art du théâtre, intended as a manual for amateur actors, was François Riccoboni's only book on acting. It advanced the notion that actors do not feel the emotions they portray on stage but rather imitate so skilfully the external signs of feelings that the audience will presume them emotionally affected (Riccoboni, 1750: 36–37). In this consists the actor's power of expression: in making the spectator feel what he does not. Published in 1750, *L'Art du théâtre* employs a series of arguments in favour of the unfeeling actor which are analogous to those suggested by *Premier*; for instance: the incompatibility between the actor's emotional arousal and her control over the performance (Riccoboni, 1750: 37–38), the actor's labour being physically rather than emotionally demanding (Riccoboni, 1750: 41), actors knowing that they do not feel but wanting to keep it as their secret (Riccoboni, 1750: 36–37). They are intriguing coincidences, if they are indeed coincidences rather than simply borrowings on Diderot's part; as has been suggested, the Paradoxe appears to be a development of the ideas put forth in *L'Art du théâtre* (De Luca, 2015: 123). Yet there are also distinct divergences between Riccoboni's book and the *Paradoxe*, not least the fact that *L'Art du théâtre* is a manual on acting, while the *Paradoxe* is a philosophical dialogue focused on a discussion of sensibility, which it extends to wider contexts. Besides, *Premier*'s expansion of the formulation of the unfeeling actor to epitomize a cynical personality, with the ensuing negative moral judgment, is all Diderot's and completely extraneous to Riccoboni's text.

The allusion to Riccoboni in the *Paradoxe* is rather casual, and so is the reference to his supposed opponent, Sainte-Albine; nonetheless it evokes an association between the two authors which is strikingly relevant, if unexplored. Although he does not mention it in his treatise, Riccoboni had read *Le Comédien*, and had written *L'Art du théâtre* partly as a refutation of some of its principles (De Luca, 2015), as *Premier* himself hints at. But the interconnections between these authors extend even further. Not only is Sainte-Albine's book genetically linked to the *Garrick* (Valentino, 2011; Harriman-Smith, 2015), but both his and Riccoboni's essays are part of a group of texts which examine the art of the actor in a cross-referential context. What I take to represent the direct and indirect references to the *Paradoxe* – that fertile ground of discussion without which the *Paradoxe* would be, I think, unconceivable, notwithstanding the genius of its author – harbour a yet unexplored goldmine. Describing the cross-referential nature of these works provides an amazing picture of the coherent development of ideas on the art of the actor in the eighteenth century.

Genetic and trans-European links

Notably, the *Paradoxe*'s referencing establishes an affinity between *Le Comédien* and the *Garrick*, whose depth was most likely unknown to Diderot himself as well as to other protagonists of the time. As first reconstructed by William Archer (1888) and further clarified by recent scholarly research (Valentino, 2011), these two treatises are joined by a direct genetic link. Pierre Rémond de Sainte-Albine, a French journalist and author of a few plays, first published *Le Comédien* in 1747, but the book, given its success, saw a second, augmented and definitive edition in 1749. This second edition was the subject, as early as 1750, of a translation and adaptation into English in a book called *The Actor: A Treatise on the Art of Playing. Interspersed with Theatrical Anecdotes, Critical Remarks on Plays, and Occasional Observations on Audiences*. This work, published anonymously, was authored by John Hill, an amateur actor, literary critic and botanist. Hill's work was also successful, judging from the fact that it was published in a number of re-editions, culminating in the latest one of 1755 (Valentino, 2011). Whilst the 1750 version is an almost faithful translation of Sante-Albine's treatise, the 1755 one differs substantially from the original. The title itself, *The Actor: or a Treatise on the Art of Playing. A New Work, Written by the author of the former, and Adapted to the Present State of the Theatres* (hereafter cited as *The Actor*), announces it as a new work. In fact, the organization of the material loses the structure of divisions and chapters as inherited by *Le Comédien*, develops further its theoretical content, and features the notable addition of copious illustrative examples taken from the contemporary English acting practice. As a last transition, Sticotti's *Garrick* is a loose translation of the 1755 edition of *The Actor*, which generally keeps to the structure and content of the source text, preserving the examples taken from the English stage. The main deviation from John Hill's book, besides the restyling of some of the passages, is the addition of notes which contain the translator's comments, as well as examples of acting practice taken from the contemporary French stage, mostly the *Comédie Française*. Sticotti's book too enjoyed a great success, with at least three editions appearing within three years (Archer, 1888: 18).

Diderot was almost certainly unaware of the derivation of the *Garrick* from *Le Comédien*; and it is plausible that Sticotti himself was ignorant that his French translation of Hill's book rooted back into a French treatise. Nevertheless, this critical line of connection highlights that the *Garrick* is the outcome of a congruent discourse on acting which had developed across different European heritages. There are therefore reasons to refute one of *Premier*'s objections against the *Garrick*: that is, the book's absurd pretence to prescribe rules of acting which are presumed to apply to such different theatrical cultures as the French and English ones (Diderot, 1883: 5–6). What Diderot did not know is that the views on acting expressed in the *Garrick* had been passed across the Channel precisely because they had been thought to be applicable beyond national boundaries, and examples from the French and English theatres had gradually been incorporated as proof of their transnational relevance. Moreover, the trans-European reach of their context extends to incorporate the Italian heritage of *Commedia dell'Arte*, which was part of the theatrical culture of eighteenth-century France. It is significant, but rarely noticed, that Michel Sticotti, the author of the *Garrick*, makes a specific reference to François Riccoboni's views on acting in one of his notes to the book. In the note (Sticotti, 1770: 148–149, note 'n') he explains that two renowned actors, who have both written on acting, have expressed contrary opinions 'on a rather important point', namely whether the actor's emotional arousal is the perfection of her art or rather its undoing. The two actors, in Archer's (1888: 11) terms an emotionalist and an anti-emotionalist, are no less than Luigi and François Riccoboni. Although Sticotti does not spell out their full names and calls them respectively Mr R. L. and Mr R. F., it is not unconceivable that Diderot might have become aware of François Riccoboni's treatise precisely through this note in the *Garrick.*

Sticotti's mention of the Riccobonis' opinions was based on solid acquaintance, given that they were all members of the company running the *Comédie Italienne*, the Italian theatre in Paris sponsored by the French monarchy. Luigi Riccoboni, a renowned Italian actor-manager within the *Commedia dell'Arte* tradition, was operating a reformation of theatre in Italy when, in 1716, he was endowed by his patron, the Duke of Modena, on behalf of the Regent of France, Philippe d'Orléans, to re-open the Italian theatre in Paris. The old *Comédie Italienne* had been previously shut down by Louis XIV in 1697, with the shameful expulsion of all its actors (Clarke, 1992). In forming his company in Italy, Luigi Riccoboni had recruited a young married couple, Fabio Sticotti and Ursula Astori, Michel's parents in fact. Michel, born in France, had an older brother, Antonio, to whom scholarly tradition mistakenly continues to attribute the authorship of the *Garrick* (see for instance Harriman-Smith, 2015: 83, as the latest of a long list of examples). In fact, following that practice of inaccurate referencing which equally concerns the Riccobonis, the author of the *Garrick* is referred to as Antonio Fabio, a conflation of Michel's brother and father.[2] Antonio Sticotti pursued his career as actor and playwright within the walls of the *Comédie Italienne* and in close collaboration and competition with François Riccoboni, while Michel failed his debut with the company in 1739 and went to perform first into the provinces and then abroad, including a short stay in London in 1749. Because Antonio was much better known in France, Michel's literary works, including his various theoretical works on the theatre, were, and still are, wrongly attributed to his brother (Meldolesi, 1969).[3]

Sticotti's note on the Riccobonis reveals a connection between the *Paradoxe*'s references which runs even deeper. Not only were Michel Sticotti and the Riccobonis closely associated, but the connection between Sainte-Albine and Luigi Riccoboni must also be alluded to, for the sake of completion. Sainte-Albine (1749: 1) introduces *Le Comédien* as the first attempt to establish the language and theory of the art of the actor, whose terminology and principles, he claims, have been so little developed. His claim at primacy is artfully misleading in as far as it eludes any reference to Luigi Riccoboni's contributions, in particular his *Pensées sur la Declamation*, published in 1738, an essay on oratory and acting written in French prose to make it readily accessible to a wide audience. The work enjoyed good success and was translated into English as early as 1741 (Cappelletti, 1986: 14). François Riccoboni (1750: 3–4) praised its merits in *L'Art du théâtre*. This was not mere partisanship, if the same *Pensées sur la Declamation* enthused, much later, the Russian master Stanislavski, who, it is reported, after reading the book 'trembled with excitement. "Oh, the darling, the darling!" he exclaimed in a voice of infinite tenderness, stretching out his arms as though he could actually see the old Italian actor before him and wished to press him to his heart' (Magarshack, 1950: 336–337, cited in Cappelletti, 1986: 15).

It is difficult to believe that Sainte-Albine was not aware of Luigi Riccoboni's essay, given that he was personally acquainted with its author and given his endeavour to write a treatise on the same subject. A curious dramaturgical event in the history of the *Comédie Italienne* proves the degree of familiarity between the two men. In 1716, the year of the arrival of Luigi Riccoboni's troupe in Paris, Sainte-Albine was a young intellectual participating in the fashionable literary circles which saw the birth of the first collaborations between the Italian theatre and French playwrights. The string of successes of the Italian troupe had spurred cynics and enemies to doubt the supposed improvised nature of the actors' performances. On the occasion of a particularly successful play, Sainte-Albine suggested challenging the Italian troupe to stage a scenario newly written for them and he composed the scenario *Lélio Vainqueur des Epreuves de la Constance*, which was successfully performed by the troupe without previous rehearsals (Courville, 1945: 115–117). The protagonist of the play, Lelio, was the stock character played by Luigi Riccoboni. A prominent figure of the Parisian theatrical scene in the first half of the eighteenth century, and formerly one of the most important actor-managers and playwrights of the *Commedia dell'Arte* tradition in Italy, theorist and reformer, Luigi Riccoboni[4] is the undercurrent who links together emotionalists and anti-emotionalists, including Diderot. As a final hint, suffice it to say that one of the six original scenarios that Luigi Riccoboni wrote as part of his attempted reformation of Italian comedy was the source for Goldoni's play *Il vero amico*, on which Diderot in turn based the plot of *Le Fils naturel*.

The emotionalist texts on acting

Although Luigi Riccoboni was a central protagonist of the eighteenth-century debate on acting, and closely linked with the development of the emotionalist theory, here I will concentrate on the three essays on acting which come to represent the culmination of the emotionalist position: *Le Comédien*, *The Actor* and the *Garrick*.[5] Because two of these texts are written in French and one in English, and each one is a transposition of the other, a comment on terminology is necessary, particularly for those words which are central to the discussion of acting. In the *Paradoxe*'s discussion of the unfeeling actor, the critical terms are sensibility (*sensibilité*) and judgement (*jugement*). For what concerns the first concept, the *Garrick* equally makes use of the word '*sensibilité*', which is a translation of the English word 'sensibility' employed by Hill. In *Le Comédien*, however, the word employed by Sainte-Albine and translated by Hill as 'sensibility' is '*sentiment*'. It has been claimed that when Hill translated *Le Comédien*, he possibly clarified an ambiguity present in Sainte-Albine's use of the term '*sentiment*' (Roach, 1993: 100), given that sensibility and sentiment have different meanings in English, one describing the capacity to respond to sensations, the second the sensation itself (Roach, 1993: 99). This distinction however is mistakenly applied to the eighteenth-century usage. Notably, the *Encyclopédie*[6] has one single entry for the words '*sensibilité*' and '*sentiment*', indicating their overlapping meaning. Not only 'in the moral and social vocabulary of eighteenth-century France, *sensibilité* belonged to the same family of words as *sens, sensation, sentiment, sentimental*, and *sensiblerie*' (Vila, 1998: 2), but also within eighteenth-century English literature and philosophy terms such as sensibility and sentiment were often used interchangeably (Todd, 1986: 6). A close reading of *Le Comédien* and *The Actor* shows unequivocal consistency of meaning between Sainte-Albine's use of the term '*sentiment*' and its subsequent renderings as sensibility or '*sensibilité*'.

For what concerns 'judgement', its inter-textual renditions are complicated by the fact that authors do not invariably employ one word for it, but may move between different words. For instance, Sticotti alternates between the use of '*jugement*' and '*intelligence*' to translate Hill's interchangeable terms of 'judgement' and 'understanding'. Sainte-Albine instead uses the word '*esprit*' to describe the rational element of the actor's art as opposed to '*sentiment*'. Ultimately, all these words invoke the same notion. In the entry in the *Encyclopédie*,[7] composed by Voltaire, *esprit* partakes of the wider semantic field comprising words such as *jugement* and *intelligence*. In discussing its meaning, Voltaire explains that when applied to human beings, *esprit* denotes rational thinking, as opposed to the divine *esprit* which amounts to intuition. In philosophy *esprit* is a quality of the soul and can signify a number of different mental operations such as judgement, talent, taste, discernment, intelligence and so on, and needs to be accompanied by a specifying word in order for its meaning to be precisely stipulated. The analysis of the emotionalist texts suggests that 'understanding' intended as comprising intelligence, judgement and sympathy, is an apposite modern English rendition for this concept when applied to the emotionalist formulation of the art of the actor.

Le Comédien

In his '*Avertissement de l'auteur*' prefaced to the second edition of *Le Comédien*, Sainte-Albine touches on the very question that Diderot identifies as the kernel of the art of the actor: the relationship between sensibility and judgement. In the first edition, he had maintained that the actor needs to possess much understanding (*esprit*), to which critics had raised the objection that instinct and sensibility (*instinct et sentiment*) had been the recognized principal attributes of some good contemporary actresses. In the second edition, he responds to this point of contention by an intriguing remark: that in extremely sensitive souls '*sentiment* sometimes turns into *esprit*' (Sainte-Albine, 1749: 2).[8] Sainte-Albine recognizes the difficulties in discussing this subject, given that various authors attribute divergent meanings to the same words: 'Not only some reject those maxims that others take for granted, but also the words employed are not given the same meaning' (Sainte-Albine, 1749: 5–7).[9] Diderot will briefly put this same point at the beginning of the *Paradoxe*, where he attributes the contradictory nature of ideas and opinions on the actor's art to the vagueness and lack of specificity of the language employed. As we have seen, his *Premier* will be guilty of contributing considerably to such confusion, especially for what concerns his interpretation of what sensibility entails.

The discussion of '*esprit*' and '*sentiment*' occupies most of *Le Comédien*'s first section. Although Sainte-Albine considers both to be natural endowments, he specifies that they need to be developed and refined by art (Sainte-Albine, 1749: 16). Therefore any equation between *sentiment* and instinct is deceptive. This is especially true because both *esprit* and *sentiment* concern the actor's ability to create a character which is beyond any equation with her person. *Esprit* corresponds to the actor's ability to think, to reflect – an ability without which, Sainte-Albine insists, a good actor cannot do. *Esprit* is the actor's capability for observing and distinguishing the details of her role, relating the quality and degree of the different emotions to the circumstances of her character – the 'given circumstances' later embedded in theatrical jargon by Stanislavski (1980: 50–52). The actor's ability to feel is far from enough; 'she needs to arouse her feelings no more than is appropriate and to the degree required by the circumstances' (Sainte-Albine, 1749: 21).[10] In its function to guide what in modern terms we would call the interpretation of a role, *esprit* is raised to the honours of helmsman of the actor's art: '*Esprit* is hence as necessary to the actor as the pilot to the ship. It is *esprit* that holds the rudder; it is *esprit* that directs the manoeuvres, and that shows and plans the route' (Sainte-Albine, 1749: 26).[11]

Sainte-Albine (1749: 26) concedes that a long experience of the theatre may sometimes make up for a lack of *esprit*, and he admits the possibility that a great actor playing by instinct may fortuitously provide a correct interpretation, but such success will be short-lived and soon her lack of command over her acting will become apparent. The cliché of the lack of consistency in the performance of actors who play by instinct will be cited by all the essays originating from *Le Comédien* and is to be found in the *Paradoxe* itself. Diderot will condemn acting by instinct on the very same basis on which the emotionalists, from Sainte-Albine to Sticotti, had done, and yet he will not admit to the consonance of his position with theirs. On the contrary, Diderot will make his censure of actors who play by instinct appear to be a justification of his crusade against the emotionalists, his attitude only serving to highlight that some of the *Paradoxe*'s arguments against the emotionalist position are unjustified and frankly mistaken. As a final attempt at clarifying the contentious point of whether *esprit* should be considered an important component of the actor's art and why it has been often dismissed, Sainte-Albine (1749: 28) offers the explanation of the different connotations that the word carries. In certain social gatherings *esprit* may signify 'wit', but such meaning is the most misleading if applied to the type of *esprit* that he requires of the actor: not a vain and superficial display, but a deep and useful form of understanding. Notably, Sainte-Albine is attempting to shed some light on that imprecision of language which both he and later Diderot will identify as one of the causes of the confusion surrounding this subject.

If the discussion of *esprit* was already advancing the argument in the direction of explaining the attributes of the actor's art, Sainte-Albine's effort with regards to *sentiment* is even more thorough. *Sentiment* is not the actor's temperamental predisposition to soft feelings and easy tears, although this may be of use to tragic actors, as much as a natural predisposition to cheerfulness is useful to comic actors. 'The meaning of this word has much more scope, and it defines, in actors, the ease of making the various emotions, to which humans are susceptible, follow one another in their soul' (Sainte-Albine, 1749: 31–32).[12] *Esprit* and '*cœur*' (*sentiment*) of an actor need to become 'like soft wax' ('*comme une cire molle*') (Sainte-Albine, 1749: 32), to allow themselves all the modifications appropriate to the interpretation of the role according to the author's text. This is the quality that an actor cannot be in want of. Although this exposition appears in a chapter dedicated to *sentiment*, Sainte-Albine does not draw such a sharp distinction between the function of *sentiment* as opposed to that of *esprit*. As the theory will get elaborated by Hill in his 1755 edition of *The Actor*, the quintessential quality of the actor's art will be eventually identified as *esprit*, or rather 'understanding' or 'judgement' (the words used in the English translation and adaptation of *Le Comédien*), while sensibility will be demoted to second place. It is not so much that *The Actor*, by emphasizing the role of judgement, represents an intermediate position between Sainte-Albine and Diderot, as has been claimed (Harriman-Smith, 2015: 90). It is rather more correct to say that the English adaptation enhances the value of judgement as compared to sensibility to an even greater degree, but that the importance of judgement in the actor's art had never been disputed by its French source either.

Taking up a notion that he has already offered under the chapter dedicated to *esprit*, Sainte-Albine assumes that the aim of the actor is to display 'the kind and degree of feeling' ('*l'espece et le dégré de sentiment*') (Sainte-Albine, 1749: 38) which she achieves through her ability not only to take on the different emotions but also to move swiftly from one to the other. Such ability will be much more easily exercised, says Sainte-Albine, if the actor does not allow any distraction by her personal feelings, and a tendency not to be affected by her own pains or joys will enhance the quality of her performance. The obvious implications of this conceptualization are that the actor's ease in feeling the character's emotions (of the right kind and degree) is in inverse proportion with her inclination to be sentimental with regards to her own affairs. This formulation is particularly revealing of the distinction between Diderot's and the emotionalists' notions of sensibility. For the emotionalists, sensibility has nothing to do with the actor's personal feelings; on the contrary, the actor's sensibility has the function of arousing the character's feelings in the actor, its operations being greatly facilitated if the actor stirs away from her own personal feelings.

Following the discussion of *esprit* and *sentiment*, there is another quality which Sainte-Albine identifies as essential to the actor's art, what he calls '*feu*', or fire, and which represents the actor's power of expression. *Feu* allows the actor to express effectively those character's emotions that she has correctly identified with *esprit* and reproduced within herself with *sentiment*, accomplishing thereby her final aim to affect the spectator's feelings. Again, the description of *feu* is accompanied by the clarification that the actor's emotions need to correspond to the quality and degree required by the expressive demands of the characterization of her role within the intentions of the play (Sainte-Albine, 1749: 44). On the other hand, the random expression of emotions unguided by *esprit* denotes lack of *feu*, and Sainte-Albine again clarifies a terminological inconsistency: what others have erroneously identified as instances in which an actor had too much *feu* were in fact situations in which actors had arbitrarily moved away from expressing the character's emotions and into wrongly expressing their own personal feelings, with 'unreason and awkwardness' (*déraison et maladresse*) (Sainte-Albine, 1749: 46). Sainte-Albine, and Hill after him, call 'fire' the actor's expressive power (Wasserman, 1947: 270), that is, her ability to affect the audience through her feelings. Rooting back into classical rhetoric, the orator's or actor's 'fire' is intended as her capacity to transfer – or project, to use a modern term – her feelings into the audience as if by contagion, like the fire spreads from object to object through proximity (Vicentini, 2011: 19). In this sense, 'fire' represents a concrete means of communication between actors and audience, without the interposition of a mediating psychic function such as the imagination. This idea accords, as we shall remember, with Hume's (in Csengei, 2011: 40–41) notion that sympathy is founded on the interpersonal transmission of feelings. What is however distinct about the emotionalist formulation of 'fire' is that the actor needs to be able to emanate, or transfer, not her personal feelings, but those of the character. *Feu* must abide by the same rules of *sentiment*, namely, be under the control of *esprit*, to avoid the spectator that displeasing sensation which is mistakenly attributed to 'too much *feu*', and must instead be construed as caused by 'too little *feu*': as far as *feu* represents the ability to express the character's feelings in their right kind and degree, there cannot be too much of it.

It could seem extremely puzzling that a theory so much at pain to emphasize the use of intelligent insight and controlled expression of feelings against arbitrariness, personalism and instinct may have lent itself to be so much misunderstood. And yet there is an important reason why. Following the exposition of these principles, in the second part of the book (*Livre second*) Sainte-Albine proceeds indeed to discuss other topics that contradict the earlier remarks, in particular with his requirement that actors who will play the roles of lovers be lovers in their personal life, or that tragic actors be noble in spirit. Furthermore, as a legacy of the rhetoric tradition, *Le Comédien* stands by rules of propriety ('*le sentiment fin des convenances*', Sainte-Albine, 1749: 21), which will necessarily be called upon to limit the actor's expression even at the expense of truth (Fumaroli, 1993: 704). Sainte-Albine's intention to write a practical manual for the use of actors, rather than a philosophical essay, contributed to the perpetuation of clichés (Meldolesi, 1969: 160), which were adopted by the translations and adaptations of *Le Comédien*. Unfortunately, this circumstance crippled the significance that these texts could have held for the theory of acting, while leaving to the *Paradoxe* the merit of having focused the discussion on the specific dilemma of the function of feeling in the art of the actor. In the resolution of this dilemma lies the crucial divergence between the emotionalists' and Diderot's contentions, because Diderot, following or paralleling François Riccoboni, will dispute the existence of that continuity between the spectator's and the actor's emotional experience, by which the emotionalists abide.

Despite maintaining that the actor needs to be able to manipulate her sensibility sheltered from the influence of any personal or spontaneous feelings, Sainte-Albine positively rejects the possibility that this psychic operation may equate to simulation. He imagines being confronted with the objection that because certain actresses are so good at feigning with their lovers in private, then they must be equally good at feigning on the stage (Sainte-Albine, 1749: 39). His answer is that in personal life a lover may have a certain vested interest in being tricked and the lover's vanity will push him to believe more easily in the actress's love. On the other hand, spectators hold it more to their interest to find out those actors who feign, as an audience wants to be tricked through the theatrical illusion, but not too grossly. The spectator's vanity pushes him to disbelieve rather than to believe, and he will reject any gross attempt at feigning. A potent anchor to the rules of rhetoric, the continuity between the actor's and the spectator's emotional experience is re-affirmed.

The Actor

The treatise of *The Actor* merits special attention because of the important function it serves in the transposition of ideas on acting between France and England, and for representing the substantial link between *Le Comédien* and the *Paradoxe* (Valentino, 2011). In the introduction to the 1755 edition of *The Actor*, Hill makes a considerable effort in explaining the rationale for his publication, so helping to clarify some of the questions left open by *Le Comédien*. Hill (1755: 2–3) takes pain to specify that the treatise has been written for the benefit of both actors and spectators, differently from Sainte-Albine, who had only fleetingly mentioned his target audience and identified it principally with actors. This extension of address to spectators constitutes an important innovation because it is grounded in the acknowledgement of the tight link between the actor's performance and the audience's response. Here the effect that the audience has on the actor, and its implications for acting, come under scrutiny: the audience's judgement is considered instrumental to the advancement of the actor's art, because, as Hill (1755: 2) points out, when the audience judges badly, bad acting is encouraged and real talent may be lost or remain underdeveloped. The rules set out in the book should hence contribute to the improvement of acting not only by instructing actors on 'how they advance toward it' but also by instructing audiences when to dispense their applause and when their censure.

The emphasis that Hill places on the spectators' judgement amounts to an acknowledgement that although actors put their spell on the audience, spectators are not entirely enchanted during a performance: their faculty of judgement remains active alongside their submission to the theatrical illusion. Although eighteenth-century emotionalists and anti-emotionalists, including Diderot, do not doubt that the audience's experience at the theatre entails emotional identification with the characters' feelings, the theatrical illusion does not obliterate their rational faculties or their self-awareness. In his *Preface to Shakespeare* of 1765 Samuel Johnson (1765: 14) affirms: 'The truth is, that the spectators are always in their senses, and know, from the first act to the last, that the stage is only a stage, and that the players are only players'. In William Archer's (1888: 150) terms, the spectator could be said to exercise his dual consciousness. The spectator's capacity for judgement has therefore at least two scopes: it is the proof that emotional identification is not equivalent to the spectator forgetting who or where he is, namely that he has not fallen mad, and it is also the means through which the audience can exert their power over actors, praising or censuring according to their taste. If the art of the actor is of consequence to spectators, then it is only reasonable that they should have a vested interest in overseeing its quality. Importantly, their praise and censure are supposed to signal to actors the way towards improving their practice, therefore effectively implying that the art of the actor can be learnt.

In point of fact, the whole of the first chapter of *The Actor* is dedicated to emphasizing the need for study in the actor's art. As an evolution of the ideas found in *Le Comédien*, the emphasis falls on the prominence of artistic endeavour rather than innate talent. Hill believes that acting depends so much on acquired skills, that while natural talents are important for principal players, most actors can just do with the sole contribution of art: 'while those [the capital performers] improve and perfect themselves by art, these [the others] may form themselves entirely upon it' (Hill, 1755: 4). Garrick is described as the paradigmatic example of the talented actor who cultivates with 'indefatigable assiduity' (Hill, 1755: 5) the talents that nature has endowed him with. Garrick, celebrated in *The Actor* for his dedication to studying his art, shall also be Diderot's example of the perfection of skilful acting, another point of consonance between Diderot and his alleged adversaries which invalidates once again Diderot's contention that they supposedly praise a form of acting squarely opposed to his. In fact, like it was for *Le Comédien*, the emphasis on the use of intelligence leads *The Actor* to the condemnation of spontaneity and instinct: when acting 'is ungoverned and undirected we may admire a flight, or stare at some unexpected stroke, but after that we are disgusted' (Hill, 1755: 7). This passage, which runs from Sainte-Albine, through Hill and Sticotti into Diderot nearly unaltered, here is taken to more extreme consequences with the condemnation of acting by instinct as carrying the risk of extravagance, of which nothing can be more contemptible. In a way, the mistakes of a great natural talent who acts without art are less tolerable than the mistakes of untalented actors. 'Insipidity is the general character of inferior performers; and extravagance is too much that of the superior ones' (Hill, 1755: 8). While uneducated audiences may be unable to discern, sophisticated spectators will be offended by both these faults, and their 'censure falls almost entirely upon the superior class: they pity what the others cannot help, but they condemn in these what their judgement ought to have taught them to avoid' (Hill, 1755: 8).

Extravagance derives from the lack of judgment which leaves sensibility unleashed, while sensibility must be regulated by understanding in order to establish the basis of good acting. As already endorsed by *Le Comédien*, there is an indissoluble link between sensibility and judgement in the actor's art, a notion very much at odds with the absolute opposition established by *Premier* between sensibility and judgement. And *The Actor* brings the argument full circle back to the effect on the spectator. The extravagance of uncontrolled sensibility not only induces the spectator to advance a negative judgement on the actor, but disgusts the spectator by forcing itself upon him and leaving him with a sense of untruthfulness and displeasure (Hill, 1755: 11). It is in fact this effect on the spectator's sensibility that is ultimately the cause of the spectator's negative judgement. In both actors and spectators, thought and feeling, judgement and sensibility are at their best when they work in unison. As spectators, says Hill (1755: 10), 'we feel, as if they were our own, the sentiments and passions represented by a good writer, and animated by a performer who has judgement and genius'. Although sensibility and judgement have both got a place in *The Actor*'s theory, judgement clearly surpasses sensibility in the re-worked edition of the treatise and the actor's art becomes 'a science, and is to be studied as a science' (Hill, 1755: 12). What could be more opposed to Diderot's pretension that Sticotti, faithful translator of *The Actor*, glorifies acting based on natural instinct?

After taking great pain to explain the supremacy of judgement and art over sensibility and nature in Chapter I, *The Actor* dedicates the whole of Chapter II to illustrating the importance of understanding (or judgement), with lots of examples taken from the contemporary English stage. But what is it that the actor needs to judge or understand? Again, it is Hill who clarifies and extends insights already mentioned by Sainte-Albine. The actor is expected to understand the ideas contained in the text which she receives from the author. These ideas are not descriptions of the states of mind of the characters, but rather such states of mind are what the actor needs to derive from studying the text: 'Here it is that the greatest discernment of an actor is shewn, in understanding the intent of the author; and his highest judgement in representing the temper of his mind as the other intended'

(Hill, 1755: 14). Understanding serves the purpose of distinguishing the passions in nature and degree according to the given circumstances (Hill, 1755: 29) but also to mark the transitions from one to the other (Hill, 1755: 37). This skilful activity will eventually lead the actor to the portrayal of feelings which will solely ring true to the audience, an important purpose of her effort if the stage is to represent the human mind (Hill, 1755: 20). The actor is ultimately at the service of truth, and although she is at the service of the playwright's text, she also has a duty to enhance those ideas where the author has been incomplete, becoming 'in some degree an author' herself (Hill, 1755: 31). Retaining the parallel argument of *Le Comédien*, Hill asks whether acting by imitation may 'supply the place of understanding' (Hill, 1755: 21) and refutes such proposition more definitely than Sainte-Albine, adding the example of Garrick as proof of an actor who is so great and so original that it would be impossible to suppose that his greatness is due to imitation. Moreover, the supposition of imitation at the basis of acting would impede any scope of advancement in the discipline, because any bad practice would be perpetuated indefinitely.

The chapter dedicated to 'understanding' already contains mention of sensibility, to which Chapter III will be dedicated. This is because, as it should be evident by now, understanding and sensibility are interconnected, and their discussion needs to proceed interwoven. As it was for understanding, the discussion of sensibility is also redundant at times, with the same ideas reiterated in various manners. Such ideas are similar to those already asserted by *Le Comédien*, the main difference being that in *The Actor* sensibility loses the parity with understanding and is demoted to second position, becoming the next most important requisite for the actor's art (Hill, 1755: 48). Following the rule of the Greek orator, Hill (1755: 49) does not question 'that whatever passion we would raise by our discourse in others, we must first feel ourselves [. . .] The disposition to receive those impressions by which our own passions are affected, is this quality of sensibility' which allows the actor's heart to be 'as the shapeless wax pliable' and 'ready to be moulded' at her pleasure (Hill, 1755: 59). Hill (1755: 51–52) specifies that men and actors may possess sensibility in variable degrees and that its operations do not depend per se on understanding, as sensibility can manifest in actors independently of judgement; but according to the emotionalists, these instances drive to the extravagance that displeases the audience. As already emphasized by Sainte-Albine, sensibility unregulated by understanding runs the risk of misleading actors into exhibiting their own personal feelings: 'these people make a mistake when they suppose this is an excellence: The passion they exhibit is their own, and not that of the character' (Hill, 1755: 34). The only true sensibility is a 'ductility of mind', which grants the actor the ability to feel and express all emotions, and to make quick transitions between different emotions. Consequently, the actor's heart needs to be free of any personal emotion, to be ready to receive those required by the interpretation of the character (Hill, 1755: 61).

In keeping with *Le Comédien*, Hill (1755: 75) specifies that sensibility should not be conceived as restricted to 'the tender and melancholy passions', a restriction that Diderot (1883: 56) seems to apply in the *Paradoxe*, interpreting sensibility as the tendency 'to being upset, to tears, to faintings, to rescues, to flights, to exclamations'. In any case, it is Diderot's (1883: 55) outright refusal to regard sensibility as the ability to understand human nature in its infinite forms and to receive all the emotions, which makes his theory absolutely at variance with the emotionalist one. As a matter of fact, *The Actor* defines sensibility as a 'disposition to be affected by the passions which plays are intended to excite' (Hill, 1755: 48) and therefore an accomplished actor should be equally able to feel and express all emotions, and to make quick transitions between different emotions. Again, among the many examples taken from the English stage, Garrick stands out as the actor who 'runs from one passion into another, with a consummate ease' (Hill, 1755: 69), a quality that Diderot had the opportunity to witness at first hand, as *Premier* recounts in the *Paradoxe* (Diderot, 1883: 38). Although qualities of sensibility and understanding may often be disjoint in actors, it is sensibility piloted by understanding (the helmsman according to the metaphor in *Le Comédien*) which makes great acting: 'What we should wish in the perfect player is, that he has all the sensibility [. . .] and yet all the command of himself necessary to regulate its emotions' (Hill, 1755: 53–54). What Hill classifies as the perfect player is an actor who comprises in herself the emotional expression that in the *Paradoxe* Diderot assigns to Mademoiselle Dumesnil and the rational control that he grants to Mademoiselle Clairon. The great actor 'has both in such a degree, that while the judgement regulates the sensibility, the sensibility animates, enlivens, and inspires the understanding' (Hill, 1755: 58).

It will come as no surprise that Hill (1755: 77) preserves Sainte-Albine's argument against the proposition that an actor be effective in feigning emotions, as much as a deceitful mistress can feign love:

> The lover is desirous to believe the lady is fond of him, and therefore he is easily made to receive the pretence of such a fondness: but an audience are unbiased; they look with eyes of impartiality; they will not allow what does not exist.

Keeping to the rule of the Greek orator, Hill (1755: 92) maintains that 'what the actor himself does not feel, he will never make the audience feel, tho' he copy ever so perfectly the best player who ever pronounced a sentence'. This is the true measure of the schism between Diderot and what he considers his opponents: if excessive and unregulated sensibility is the enemy of good acting, and understanding is the first quality of an actor, it is the cooperation between understanding and sensibility which leads the actor to her 'paradox': that she may feel while being in control of her feelings. Diderot's notion of the paradox of the actor entails instead that no feeling at all must occupy the psyche of the great actor.

Garrick ou les acteurs anglois

Because the *Garrick* is principally a translation of the final edition of *The Actor*, mostly its content is analogous to that of its source. In keeping with the remarks found in *The Actor*, the *Garrick* grants the audience the ability to respond to a performance both by submitting to the emotional identification with the characters and by being a sober judge of the actors' performance, from which follows the necessity to educate the spectators' taste to make them active contributors to the enhancement of the actor's art. The actor's first quality is, in accordance with *The Actor*, identified with '*intelligence*', *sensibilité* being the second most important: 'Among all the natural qualities of the actor, a propitious understanding is, without doubt, the most necessary' (Sticotti, 1770: 25).[13] The interplay between *sensibilité* and *jugement* (or *intelligence*, given that the two words are used interchangeably) is also expressed as the intertwining of nature and art, again following an idea already present in *The Actor*: 'art taken to its extreme becomes nature [. . .] great actors never abandon it; they raise from that base a structure, so to speak, more natural than nature itself' (Sticotti, 1770: 10).[14] Sticotti further underscores this point in one of his notes: it is part of the actor's creative function to amend the author's possible affectation or lack of truthfulness through a performance which is natural and simple: the actor's study and art are put to the service of a performance which is devoid of artfulness, but appears instead more natural than nature itself. Garrick is unsurprisingly given as the quintessential example of the actor who has perfected his art through study; whoever thinks that Garrick is a 'born actor' is grossly mistaken: his excellence can only be borne out of tireless study (Sticotti, 1770: 8). Sticotti's text demonstrates once more what a scholar has rightly called Diderot's 'considerably reductive reading of Sticotti' (Vicentini, 2012: 19). The only way by which Diderot could justify his spiteful disapproval of Sticotti's book was if no one else read it and relied solely on his word. And this seems to be what mostly happened.

In another note to the text, close to the passage which states: 'The art of the theatre is a science, thus it is to be studied as a science' (Sticotti, 1770: 19),[15] Sticotti (1770: 44–45)[16] emphasizes that sensibility directed by judgement is the guiding principle of the actor to express all passions, in all circumstances, and according to their infinite variety:

> Some actors are seen crying when they should be angry. Here it is not about questioning how much sensibility they have, but how they should govern it. [. . .] It is greatly mistaken to imagine that such easy tears are an advantage; the weeping disposition is often that of the actor, not that of the character.

Predictably, sensibility is understood as disjointed from the actor's personal emotions and at the service of expressing those of the character. As it was for Sainte-Albine and Hill, and perhaps even more so, Sticotti cannot conceive of acting as deprived of feeling. In one of his notes, in which he reinforces *The Actor*'s principle that acting could never be based on imitation, he calls acting 'an art of feeling' (*un art de sentiment*) (Sticotti, 1770: 30, note 'c'). Even if faithfully keeping to his source as a translator, it appears that in his comments to the text, he undertakes to restore the emphasis on sensibility. In another note, he states that actors enter the stage impromptu and the quality of their performance greatly depends on the transitory state of their mind and body at the time; thus, even if they are the most accomplished and they have prepared their part, they cannot control the final result of their playing (Sticotti, 1770: 40, note 'g'). Sticotti's heritage of actor of the *Commedia dell'Arte* tradition weighs on his temptation to compensate for the supposedly absolute influence of judgement on the actor's art, most likely providing Diderot with that rationale for his invective, which he would not have found in *The Actor*.

A new theory of acting

Despite their clichés and inconsistencies, the emotionalist texts present a coherent theory of acting. Examining these texts closely allows not only to confute Diderot's perfunctory appraisal of their content and import, but also, and most importantly, to unearth a systematic theory of acting alternative to that found in the *Paradoxe*. There are two main levels at which Diderot's notion of the paradoxical actor and the emotionalist one differ profoundly: their reading of sensibility and their opinion about the relationship between sensibility and judgement. The emotionalist definition of sensibility is squarely opposed to that of the *Paradoxe*. If for *Premier* sensibility was the self-referential quality of expressing one's own feelings, for the emotionalists it is the ability to arouse in oneself and express the emotions of the character. In order to attain this purpose, the actor must steer away from her own personal feelings so that the operations of her sensibility are not disturbed by these. Far from being a solipsistic process, sensibility is the skill and attitude to receive the feelings of the other. The actor arouses the character's feelings in herself in order to express them for the audience. For the emotionalists, sensibility is tightly associated with the actor's fire, namely her ability to share and communicate feelings with spectators. Horace's principle that it is the orator's emotional arousal which causes the corresponding emotional involvement in the spectator is abided by. As William Archer's (1888) respondents had confirmed, most great actors believed that their emotional arousal was their most powerful tool of communication with the audience. But as the emotionalists are at pains to explain, fire is the complementary side to sensibility and it does not pertain to the expression of the actor's personal feelings. Through her fire, the actor infects spectators with the same emotional identification with the character that she is experiencing. The character stands for the 'emotional field' (Bion, 1984: 146) – to anticipate a psychoanalytic concept – through which audience and actors share and communicate feelings.

The emotions expressed through the character's interpretation are of a special kind. The absolute opposition between sensibility and judgment endorsed by the *Paradoxe* is inadmissible for the emotionalists. Not that they absolutely refuse the idea of actors in whom sensibility and judgement operate at the exclusion of each other; such actors exist, but they are poor at their art and displease and disgust spectators. The essence of competent acting lies in a dynamic relationship between sensibility and judgement: the first enlivens, the second regulates the actor's emotional identification with the character's feelings (Hill, 1755: 58). The art of the actor is not grounded in a dissociation between feelings and understanding, nor in a dual consciousness based on the ability to keep personal and character's feelings apart. It consists in the acquired capability to integrate feeling and understanding of the character's emotions. It is therefore at the service of the feelings of another. The stage, as Hill (1755: 20) puts it, must represent the human mind, and the actor's art is at the service of such representation. In this sense, Diderot's and the emotionalists' praise of Garrick as the supreme actor is founded on radically different conceptions. It puzzles Diderot how Garrick could possibly feel so many different emotions in such a short space of time and simultaneously express them effectively; he therefore must resort to dismissing Garrick's own assertion that he feels when he acts, and attributes his skill to a physical mastery of imitation of external signs of emotions. For the emotionalists, instead, Garrick's virtuosity does not need to be explained by a dissociation of the mind's control over the body from the experience of feeling; on the contrary, it is because Garrick – to borrow a metaphor from Artaud (2010: 93) – is an athlete of emotional expression that he can attain such excellent results in performance: he understands while he feels and he feels while he understands. His knowledge of emotions encompasses their expression by the body and concurrent understanding by the mind.

As I will show in the next chapter, psychoanalysis has described the psyche's ability to integrate emotions and understanding, as one of the most basic functions of mental development. This primary operation takes place at the boundaries between unconscious and conscious psychic activity, and it is therefore difficult to characterize. Because psychoanalysis focuses on unconscious mental processes, its window on the mind places it in an ideal position to capture the essence of the interplay between emotions and understanding.

Notes

1 In: Correspondance littéraire, philosophique et critique de Grimm et de Diderot, depuis 1753 jusqu'en 1790. Nouvelle édition. Tome septième, 1770–1772, p. 103, note 2, Paris: Furne et Ladrange (1829).

2 This is partly justified by the fact that Antonio took over Fabio's theatrical roles at his father's death and, by tradition, also inherited his first name (Meldolesi, 1969).

3 Michel Sticotti is also the author of other theoretical works, wrongly attributed to his elder brother Antonio Fabio, including: *Avis d'un comédien à sa fille*; *Epître à Monsieur Diderot sur la défense de continuer le Dictionnaire encyclopédique*; *Le sauvage en contradiction* (an invective against Rousseau); *Dictionnaire des passions, des vertues et des vices ou recueil des meilleurs Morceaux de morale pratique tirés des auteurs anciens & modernes, étrangers & nationnaux* (Meldolesi, 1969).

4 Between 1728 and 1743, Luigi Riccoboni wrote a copious number of works on the history and theory of the theatre, most in French, some in Italian; besides the *Pensées sur la Declamation*, these are: *Dell'Arte Rappresentativa, Discorso della commedia all'improvviso, Dissertation sur la tragédie moderne, Observations sur la comédie et sur le génie de Molière, Histoire du théâtre italien, Réflexions historiques et critiques sur les différens théâtres de l'Europe, De la Réformation du Théâtre.*

5 Given that there are more than one editions for each of these works, I have chosen to refer to: the second edition of *Le Comédien* published in 1749, which has four additional chapters as compared to the first one and presents a few corrections that the author accepted following the comments on his first edition of 1747; the 1755 edition of *The Actor*, given that the 1750 edition is merely a translation of *Le Comédien*; the second augmented edition of the *Garrick*, the only one which is extant as far as I am aware.

6 In *Encyclopédie, ou dictionnaire raisonné des sciences, des arts et des métiers, par une société de gens de lettres. Mis en ordre & publié par M. Diderot de l'Académie des Sciences et Belles-Lettres de Prusse, et quant à la partie mathématique, par M. d'Alembert de l'Académie royale des Sciences de Paris, de celle de Prusse et de la Société royale de Londres.* 1751–1772, Vol. 15, pp. 38–52, Paris: Briasson, David, Le Breton, Durand. Accessed on the web via *The Making of the Modern World.*

7 In *Encyclopédie, ou dictionnaire raisonné des sciences, des arts et des métiers, par une société de gens de lettres. Mis en ordre & publié par M. Diderot de l'Académie des Sciences et Belles-Lettres de Prusse, et quant à la partie mathématique, par M. d'Alembert de l'Académie royale des Sciences de Paris, de celle de Prusse et de la Société royale de Londres.* 1751–1772, Vol. 5, pp. 972–976, Paris: Briasson, David, Le Breton, Durand. Accessed on the web via *The Making of the Modern World.*

8 'le sentiment devient quelquefois esprit'.

9 'Non seulement les uns rejettent des maximes que les autres donnent pour constants, mais on n'attache pas les mêmes significations aux termes qu'on employe'.

10 'On veut qu'il ne se passionne qu'à propos, et dans le degré qu'exigent les circonstances'.

11 'L'esprit est donc aussi nécessaire au Comédien, que le Pilote l'est à un vaisseau. C'est l'esprit qui tient le gouvernail ; c'est lui qui dirige la manœuvre, et qui indique et calcule la route'.

12 'La signification de ce mot a beaucoup plus d'étendue, et il désigne dans les Comédiens la facilité de faire succéder dans leur ame les diverses passions, dont l'homme est susceptible'.

13 'De toutes les qualités naturelles à l'acteur, une heureuse intelligence est, sans contredit, la plus nécessaire'.

14 'l'art porté à son comble devient nature [. . .] les grands Acteurs ne l'abandonnent jamais; ils élèvent sur cette base un édifice, pour ainsi dire, plus naturel quel la nature même'.

15 'L'art du Théâtre est une science, il faut donc l'étudier comme une science'.

16 'On voit des Acteurs pleurer lorsqu'il faut se mettre en colère. Il ne s'agit pas de chercher ici combien ils ont de sensibilité, mais comment ils doivent la gouverner. [. . .] On se trompe fort d'imaginer que ces pleurs si faciles sont une beauté; la passion larmoyante est souvent celle du Comédien, non pas celle du personnage'.

Bibliography

Archer, W. (1888) *Masks or Faces: A Study in the Psychology of Acting*, London: Longmans, Green and Company.

Artaud, A. (2010) *The Theatre and Its Double*, translated by V. Corti, London: Oneworld Classics Ltd.

Bion, W. R. (1984) *Second Thoughts*, London: Karnac.

Cappelletti, S. (1986) *Luigi Riccoboni e la riforma del teatro. Dalla commedia dell'arte alla commedia borghese*, Ravenna: Longo Editore.

Clarke, J. (1992) 'The Expulsion of the Italians from the Hotel de Bourgogne in 1697', *Seventeenth Century French Studies*, vol. 14, pp. 97–117.

Courville, X. de (1945) *Luigi Riccoboni dit Lélio. II (1716–1731). L'expérience française*, Paris: Libraire E. Droz.
Csengei, I. (2011) *Sympathy, Sensibility and the Literature of Feeling in the Eighteenth Century*, Basingstoke: Palgrave Macmillan.
De Luca, E. (2015) 'Una vita nell'*Art du Théâtre*' in F.A.V. Riccoboni, *L'arte del teatro*, traduzione, introduzione e note E. De Luca, *Acting Archives Review*, Anno 5, no. 10, [Online], Available: http://www.actingarchives.it
Diderot, D. (1883) *The Paradox of Acting*, translation and annotations by Walter Herries Pollock, London: Chatto & Windus.
Fumaroli, M. (1993) 'Feu et glace: le "Comédien" de Rémond de Saint-Albine (1747), anthithèse du "Paradoxe"', *Revue d'histoire littéraire de la France*, vol. 5, pp. 702–716.
Harriman-Smith, J. (2015) 'Comédien-Actor-Paradoxe: The Anglo-French Sources of Diderot's Paradoxe sur le comédien', *Theatre Journal*, vol. 67, no. 1, pp. 83–96.
Hill, J. (1755) *The Actor: Or a Treatise on the Art of Playing: A New Work, Written by the Author of the Former, and Adapted to the Present State of the Theatres*, London: R. Griffiths.
Johnson, S. (1765) *Preface to Shakespeare*, reprint, Gloucester: Dodo Press.
Magarshack, D. (1950) *Stanislavsky: A Life*. London: Macgibbon and Kee.
Meldolesi, C. (1969) *Gli Sticotti. Comici italiani nei teatri d'Europa del Settecento*, Roma: Edizioni di Storia e Letteratura.
Riccoboni, F. (1750) *L'Art du théâtre. A Madame* ***, Paris: Simon & Giffart.
Roach, J. R. (1993) *The Player's Passion: Studies in the Science of Acting*, Ann Arbor: The University of Michigan Press.
Sainte-Albine, M.R. de (1749) *Le Comédien. Ouvrage divisé en deux parties. Nouvelle édition, augmentée et corrigée*, Paris: Desaint & Saillant.
Stanislavski, C. (1980) *An Actor Prepares*, translated by E. Reynolds Hapgood, London: Methuen.
Sticotti, M. (1770) *Garrick ou les Acteurs Anglois. Ouvrage contenant des Observations sur l'Art dramatique, sur l'Art de la Représentation, et le Jeu des Acteurs. Avec des Notes historiques et critiques, et des Anecdotes sur les différents Théâtres de Londres et de Paris*, traduit de l'anglois, seconde édition, augmentée, Paris: J.-P. Costard.
Todd, J. (1986) *Sensibility: An Introduction*, London: Methuen.
Valentino, B. (2011) 'Pierre Rémond de Sainte-Albine and John Hill. From *Le Comédien* to *The Actor*', *Acting Archives Essays: Acting Archives Review*, Supplement 12, [Online], Available: http://www.actingarchives.it
Vicentini, C. (2011) 'Theory of Acting I: Acting Theory in the Ancient World', *Acting Archives Essays: Acting Archives Review*, Supplement 1, [Online], Available: http://www.actingarchives.it
Vicentini, C. (2012) 'Theory of Acting VII. Antiemotionalism. Antoine- François Riccoboni, Lessing, Diderot', *Acting Archives Essays: Acting Archives Review*, Supplement 16, [Online], Available: http://www.actingarchives.it
Vila, A. C. (1998) *Enlightenment and Pathology: Sensibility in the Literature and Medicine of Eighteenth-Century France*, Baltimore/London: The John Hopkins University Press.
Wasserman, E. R. (1947) 'The Sympathetic Imagination in Eighteen-Century Theories of Acting', *The Journal of Acting English and Germanic Philology*, vol. 16, no. 3, pp. 264–272.

Chapter 5

Unconscious emotional processing in alpha-function

Freud's theory of ego functioning

In *Studies on Hysteria* (Freud and Breuer, 1895) and in subsequent works on the neuroses, Freud proved the relevance of unconscious mental life for explaining and for curing common neurotic disorders. But it was with the *Interpretation of Dreams* (Freud, 1900) that he proceeded to show how the unconscious was the dominant aspect of all mental life, not just of its pathology. For this reason he considered this book his most important contribution to psychology. As he declared: 'From the date of *The Interpretation of Dreams* psycho-analysis had a twofold significance. It was not only a new method of treating the neuroses but it was also a new psychology' (Freud, 1924: 200). Freud's study of depth psychology in his clinical practice led him to propose theoretical systems that could explain the functioning of the mind accounting for the unconscious as well as the conscious phenomena progressively unravelled by psychoanalysis. As he continued to revise his theories of mental functioning to make them consistent with new clinical findings, he came to realize that not only does the unconscious dominate mental life, but also that consciousness is better understood as an accidental property of psychic phenomena. In the introduction to *The Ego and the Id*, James Strachey, the eminent editor of the English *Standard Edition of the Complete Psychological Works of Sigmund Freud*, explains how Freud (1923: 7) had reached the conclusion that

> the criterion of consciousness was no longer helpful in building up a structural picture of the mind. Freud accordingly abandoned the use of consciousness in this capacity: 'being conscious' was henceforward to be regarded simply as a quality which might or might not be attached to a mental state.

The earlier Freudian model of the mind, called the topographical model, had been based on the assumption that the psyche is simply divided into an unconscious, a preconscious and a conscious area (Freud, 1915b). Conscious wishes or memories, according to this model, can become repressed under certain conditions (for example, when considered unacceptable, such as in the case of the traumatic memories of the hysterics). Through repression they become unconscious, but this does not mean that they are at rest; on the contrary repressed wishes and memories continue to push for conscious representation, and because repression counteracts this tendency, they manifest themselves under disguise, such as in a hysterical symptom. In Chapter 2 we have seen an example of this situation in Anna O.'s hydrophobia.

In the topographical model, the preconscious represents an intermediary area between the unconscious and the conscious, and it therefore regulates the communication between the two. The preconscious contains unconscious material that is very different from that contained in the unconscious. While the unconscious proper is the haven of all repressed ideas and impulses, sheltered there against the force of repression, the preconscious harbours all those unconscious contents which are not under the thumb of repression, and hence could easily become conscious, but at any given moment are not immediately present to awareness. An example would be all those memories of recent events, which can promptly be recollected at will, but which currently are not within awareness because they are of no present interest. Hence, as Freud (1933: 71) warns, it is important

> to distinguish two kinds of unconscious – one which is easily, under frequently occurring circumstances, transformed into something conscious, and another with which this transformation is difficult and takes place only subject to a considerable expenditure of effort or possibly never at all. [. . .] We call the unconscious which is only latent, and thus easily becomes conscious, the 'preconscious' and retain the term 'unconscious' for the other.

Following Freud's lesson, I make use of the term unconscious to indicate the unconscious proper, whose processes and content are not easily accessible by conscious thought and therefore pertain to an area of psychic functioning which is difficult to research and describe. This needs to be noted as a difference with other uses of the term. For instance, in the application of cognitive psychology to theorizing theatre reception, McConachie admits to the existence of unconscious aspects of spectatorship, but he tends to equate 'unconscious' with 'habitual'. An example is when he mentions cognitive blending as a psychic mechanism which occurs 'mostly below the level of consciousness' (McConachie, 2008: 42), but then he relates it back to consciousness: the spectators' 'ability to blend actors and characters into single identities depend upon mind/brain dynamics that were once partly conscious before they became habitual' (McConachie, 2008: 56). In psychoanalytic terms, the nature of such a phenomenon would be termed preconscious and have little in common with the processes characteristic of the unconscious proper.

The topographical model had the advantage of a relative simplicity and seemed to work well to explain repression, symptom formation and the relieving of symptoms in the cathartic method. However, as Freud penetrated the depth of normal and pathological mental phenomena through his extensive clinical work over two decades, he revised his theories. In particular, he came to realize that the linear explanations provided by the topographical model, despite their appeal of simplicity, did not hold true because the psyche proved to be more complex than expected. It is the seminal writing of *The Ego and the Id* (Freud, 1923) which marks the transition to what we know as Freud's structural model of the mind. The dynamic principles established in the topographical model remain valid, in as far as the relationship between conscious, preconscious and unconscious goes, and their definitions. But the structural model provides a new perspective on the mind, which is now conceptualized as divided into three different agencies: the id, the ego and the super-ego.[1] The most important innovation is that none of these agencies can be simplistically equated with consciousness. The id is entirely unconscious and the seat of the instincts; the super-ego, comprising conscience, is also largely unconscious, although part of it operates within consciousness. And, even more strikingly, the ego, the agency for awareness, conscious will and rational judgement, presents substantial unconscious portions, especially as it is the seat of repression, which is an unconscious mental operation.

Despite the emphasis on the unconscious as domineering over the psyche, Freud remains interested in consciousness, not least because it is the only modus operandi in which we can be aware of ourselves and our minds: in a way the unconscious would not be known or be recognized unless there was a consciousness which brought it to its epiphanies. On this point, he states with characteristic wit:

> And it is indeed the case that large portions of the ego and super-ego can remain unconscious and are normally unconscious. That is to say, the individual knows nothing of their contents and it requires an expenditure of effort to make them conscious. [. . .] At first we are inclined greatly to reduce the value of the criterion of being conscious since it has shown itself so untrustworthy. But we should be doing it an injustice. As may be said of our life, it is not worth much, but it is all we have. Without the illumination thrown by the quality of consciousness, we should be lost in the obscurity of depth-psychology.
>
> (Freud, 1933: 69–70)

From the psychology of impulse to the psychology of the ego

Freud's focus on the unconscious led him to investigate instinctual life extensively. In the first place, this resulted in his formulation of what is universally known as the libido theory, according to which unconscious drives, ultimately linked to a primitive sexual energy, are the foundation of all mental life, and determine the development of the child into the adult. Instincts need to negotiate their encounter with actual reality, and Freud conceptualized this as the continuous negotiation between two principles: the pleasure principle, which is the law of the instincts, and the reality principle, which must be the rule of the ego, if the ego's adaptation to reality is to be successful.

To do justice to the wide implications of libido for all mental life, Freud was aware of needing to emphasize the distinction between libido as he understood it and a restricted view of libido as genital sexuality. In his words:

> what psycho-analysis called sexuality was by no means identical with the impulsion towards a union of the two sexes or towards producing a pleasurable sensation in the genitals; it had far more resemblance to the all-inclusive and all-preserving Eros of Plato's *Symposium*.
>
> (Freud, 1925a: 218)

As he modified his model of the mind into the structural model, he also changed his theory of the instincts until he arrived at his definitive formulation, first presented in 1920 in *Beyond the Pleasure Principle*. Here Freud maintained that all human instincts are ultimately ascribable to either 'libido', the creative force of life and represented by Eros, or 'destructiveness', the annihilating force of death, ultimately leading all organisms to their dissolution, but also put at the service of the destruction of others through aggression. Thus the negotiation between pleasure and reality is complicated by the conflict between Eros and the death instinct. As Freud proceeded to recognize the ego as the negotiator of the different forces which make psychic life so complex, he gradually shifted his interest from the study of the instincts towards the study of the ego and its mechanisms. In doing so, he adumbrated many of the developments that some of his followers, and especially Melanie Klein and her circle, accomplished in psychoanalytic theory.

The relationship between the ego, the id and reality

Freud saw the ego as a specialized development of the id, which comes into being as the id is obliged to grapple with reality and adapt to it, if the baby is to survive. For example, the baby's need for food and warmth, generating from the baby's id, needs to be negotiated with the limitations that the environment, in the case of the baby especially represented by the mother, puts on the satisfaction of such needs. The way the baby adapts to such limitations will ultimately affect his development. The ego, that is, develops as the instincts meet the objects of their satisfaction or, indeed, of their frustration, in the environment. In his seminal paper on the ego, Freud (1923: 25) writes, 'It is easy to see that the ego is that part of the id which has been modified by the direct influence of the external world'. The mediation that the ego effects between the instincts of the id and external reality is also a mediation between unconscious and conscious, in as far as the external world is apprehended through sense-perceptions which are conscious, while the instincts operate at an unconscious level. It is in this way that the ego, departing from the need to manage internal drives and respond to external perceptions, enriches and develops.

Whilst the ego strives to keep control over the whole of mental life, it is not always successful. The relationship between id and ego is depicted by Freud using a metaphor which reminds us of Plato's charioteer allegory in the *Phaedrus* (246a–254e). The ego is

> in its relation to the id [. . .] like a man on horseback, who has to hold in check the superior strength of the horse [. . .] The analogy may be carried a little further. Often a rider, if he is not to be parted from his horse, is obliged to guide it where it wants to go; so in the same way the ego is in the habit of transforming the id's will into action as if it were its own.
>
> (Freud, 1923: 25)

If we borrow from Plato's allegory his depiction of the chariot being pulled by two horses, one dark and one white, who pull it in opposite directions, we come to an even more accurate image of Freud's view of the mind, with the ego having to contend with a divided id, where the creative force of Eros and the death instinct oppose each other, while the ego has to stir both in the direction indicated by the reality principle.

Identification through introjection and projection

Freud (1923: 48) suggests that both ego and super-ego (which he conceives as a specialized part of the ego) form through cycles of identification:

> Thus we have said repeatedly that the ego is formed to a great extent out of identifications which take the place of abandoned cathexes[2] by the id; that the first of these identifications always behave as a special agency in the ego and stand apart from the ego in the form of a super-ego, while later on, as it grows stronger, the ego may become more resistant to the influences of such identifications.

While he put forward a number of mechanisms through which these identifications come to be, he never brought these to bear on the formulation of a systematic and coherent theory. This will be developed instead by Melanie Klein. However he foreshadowed both projection and introjection as the two fundamental procedures underpinning identification:

> Under the dominance of the pleasure principle a further development now takes place in the ego. In so far as the objects which are presented to it are sources of pleasure, it takes them into itself, 'introjects' them (to use Ferenczi's term); and, on the other hand, it expels whatever within itself becomes a cause of unpleasure.
>
> (Freud, 1915a: 135–136)

As a note to the text indicates, 'expels' here has to be understood as equivalent to 'projects'. It is also important to note that introjection and projection are unconscious mechanisms, and the resulting identifications are equally unconscious.

Although introjection and projection are mostly described by Freud with reference to pathological states, he also describes introjection as the basis of the formation of a person's character, and sees it as especially intense during childhood (Freud, 1923: 28). His descriptions of projection are sparser. Yet, somewhat unwittingly, he gives a most interesting example of projection as a form of identification in *Beyond the Pleasure Principle* when he describes the mechanism of repetition-compulsion in the reel-game. I say unwittingly, because in this paper Freud mentions projection as a way in which the ego deals with unpleasure by projecting the unacceptable desire into an external object, but he does not connect this explicitly to identification nor to normal development. He writes:

> a particular way is adopted of dealing with any internal excitations which produce too great an increase of unpleasure: there is a tendency to treat them as though they were acting, not from the inside, but from the outside [. . .] This is the origin of projection, which is destined to play such a large part in the causation of pathological processes.
>
> (Freud, 1920: 29)

As we shall recall from Chapter 2, Freud had observed his grandson's repetitive playing with a cotton reel, throwing it away from himself and pulling it back. Freud had interpreted the game as a re-enactment. Every time his mother went away leaving the child behind for a few hours, the little boy showed little distress but engaged with the game of throwing away objects, of which the reel-game was a variant. The reel was thrown away and regained by pulling it back. As such it could represent the mother leaving the child and coming back again. But most likely, it also represented the child himself, being left behind and re-found. The little boy, losing the beloved mother through her departure, introjects her in order to avoid the pain of having lost her. Now he is unconsciously identified with her and he is the one in control of the partings and reunions. Conversely, his sense of frustrated desire for the mother and his vulnerability is projected into the cotton reel, which unconsciously becomes identified with the child himself through projection.

This example gives a very useful picture of how the ego uses unconscious identifications by introjection and projection to mediate between the instincts of the id and the necessity to adapt to reality. As Freud (1920: 16) explains in his comment on the reel-game (which I already quoted in Chapter 2):

> one gets an impression that the child turned his experience into a game for another motive. At the outset he was in a *passive* situation – he was overpowered by the experience; but, by repeating it, unpleasurable though it was, as a game, he took on an *active* part.

Freud describes the psyche as caught within a dynamic between passive and active mental processes: the ego can both be the passive recipient of instinctual forces from the id, which may risk overwhelming it, and also has a capacity for re-acting to this situation by taking an active stance towards the instincts in an attempt to master them. Through the reel-game, the child has overcome passive submission to reality, such as could have been expressed by giving in to despair and crying, and has instead engaged with an action which not only represents the reality of the mother leaving him through the surrogate object of the reel, but also offers opportunity for experimenting with such reality, insofar as the reel can be thrown away but also pulled back. In this way, the re-enactment represents the first step taken by the ego towards the reality principle, considering that it is a very basic attempt at mastering the overpowering displeasure of a frustrated instinct or need. Not least, the game permits for positions to be swapped: the reel can represent the abandoning and rejected mother, but also the abandoned child. The child, in identification with the introjected mother, and through his mastering of his actions with the reel, can experiment with the idea of sending the projected child (the reel) away. This enables the elaboration of feelings very different from those of him as the child left behind by the real mother. Significantly, these refined dramatizations of painful experiences remain unconscious.

The operations of projection and introjection will be described by Melanie Klein as cycles in which the exchange between self and other through unconscious identifications is the basic mechanism in the formation of the ego and its development throughout life. In the Kleinian theoretical system, projections and introjections act through a process of splitting of the ego, necessary if the ego can place parts of itself in others, or take parts of the others into itself. Although Freud never fully developed this concept, he recognized it in his clinical practice (Quinodoz, 2005: 151) and towards the end of his life he postulated that it is a feature of psychotic as well as neurotic disorders:

> The view which postulates that in all psychoses there is a splitting of the ego could not call for so much notice if it did not turn out to apply to other states more like the neuroses and, finally, to the neuroses themselves.
>
> (Freud, 1938: 202)

While it will have to be left to Melanie Klein to explain in a systematic way the interplay between instincts, adaptation to reality, and the mechanisms of projection and introjection, Freud had already foreshadowed it by: recognizing the importance of unconscious identification for the formation of ego and super-ego, and ultimately of character; establishing introjection and projection as the two mechanisms through which unconscious identification is effected; and noticing splitting of the ego as an unconscious process of mental life. As I will discuss in the next section, all these psychic operations – the unconscious functioning of the ego in the regulation of instincts with respect to reality, the significance of the conflict between death and life instincts, the splitting of the ego, and the mechanisms of projection and introjection as the basis for identification – became the pillars of Klein's theory of the ego's unconscious functioning. Taking Freud's structural model as a starting point, she succeeded in equipping psychoanalysis with a coherent model of ego organization through the theory of object-relations and the concept of unconscious phantasy.

Kleinian theory of object-relations

The theory of object-relations was developed principally by Melanie Klein and her collaborators, who were inspired by Freud's latest interest in the functioning of the ego with respect to its role of negotiator between instincts and reality. Klein accepted the division of all drives into the life and death instincts. She also followed Freud in the idea that the ego is fundamentally pleasure-seeking, in as much as it strives for satisfaction of the instincts and wants to get rid of pain and frustration, but it can only achieve its objective by adapting to reality. The conflicts between the life and death drives on one hand, and between the drives and the limitations of reality on the other, determine the development of the ego.

Melanie Klein started her career as a child psychoanalyst, encouraged by Sandor Ferenczi, who was one of Freud's earliest and closest disciples. During her analysis with him, he suggested she dedicate herself to the analysis of children, and thus she became one of the pioneers of child analysis (Grosskurth, 1995: 74). Although Freud (1909) had himself once been involved in the analysis of a child's phobia, in the renowned case of Little Hans, he had generally inferred his theories of child psychic development from his analysis of adults. Even in the case of Little Hans, he had met with the child only once and had de facto conducted his analysis at one remove, basing it on the observations and interventions of Hans's father, who regularly consulted with him during the period of the treatment. Klein instead developed her theories on the wealth of first-hand direct analysis of children from very young ages, including toddlers. As Hanna Segal (1989: 49) eloquently put it: 'Freud discovered the repressed child in the adult. Investigating children, Melanie Klein discovered what was already repressed in the child – namely the infant'. What allowed Klein to move psychoanalytic investigation from adults to children was the development of a specific technique, which used observation of and participation in the child's playing activity on the part of the analyst.

> Taking her cue from Freud's (1920) observation of the child's play with the reel, Melanie Klein saw that the child's play could represent symbolically his anxieties and phantasies. Since small children cannot be asked to free-associate, she treated their play in the playroom in the same way as she treated their verbal expressions, i.e. as symbolic expression of their unconscious conflicts.
>
> (Segal, 1988: 2)

In child analysis, the child is given free access to a variety of tools, such as small toys, paper and crayons, and the analyst observes his play activity in the same way as the adult's analyst would listen to her patient's free associations. The most striking aspect of Klein's technique entails that the play activities are systematically interpreted as transference situations (Klein, 1997), therefore preserving the significance of transference re-enactments for the analytic procedure and its success. While the analyst may be represented in the child's play through the use of dolls or other toys, there are times when the transference re-enactments become alive in the session, by the child actually casting the analyst in a specific role. For instance,

Klein (1929: 199) talks of a little patient, the six-year-old Erna, who would often make Klein be the child, while Erna played at being the mother or the teacher.

One interesting feature of children's play is that in it '*acting* plays a prominent part' (Klein, 1926: 135). Her extensive experience with the play technique led Klein (1929: 207) to the conclusion that personification in children's play was, in fact, the same phenomenon at the basis of transference re-enactments. This resonates with the notion that transference re-enactments may be equivalent to the Greek concept of *mimēsis* inasmuch as *mimēsis* means an innate propensity to dramatic enactments, which promotes human development. That is to say, the personifications and impersonations inherent in much of children's play, a certain meaning of *mimēsis*, and transference re-enactments, are in essence the same phenomenon. What characterizes their common nature is the way in which cycles of unconscious identifications are realized through the mental operations of projection and introjection. Klein and her close collaborators describe these unconscious mechanisms under the denomination of 'unconscious phantasy'.

Like Freud, and always preoccupied to situate her clinical and theoretical work within the legitimacy of the Freudian legacy, Melanie Klein was interested in unravelling the mysteries of the unconscious, in the belief that it was the fundamental site of psychic processes. Joan Riviere (1989:16), a Kleinian psychoanalyst and one of her close collaborators, explains:

> the unconscious is not a vestigial or rudimentary part of the mind. It is the active organ in which mental processes function; no mental activity can take place without its operation, although much modification of its primary activities normally ensues before it determines behaviour in an adult. The original primary mental activity which usually remains unconscious, we call unconscious 'phantasy'. There is, therefore, an unconscious phantasy behind every thought and every act.

By unconscious phantasy, a word purposely spelt with a 'ph' to denote its unconscious nature as opposed to 'conscious fantasy', Klein and her collaborators came to define the complex process by which psychic reality is formed through the meeting of inside impulses with their outside objects. Freud had already recognized that the interaction between internal and external reality is one of the foundations of the psyche by stating that the ego is formed to effect the negotiation between the unconscious impulses from the id and the reality that these need to confront for their satisfaction. Departing from these premises, Klein extended the psychoanalytic understanding of this process, describing systematically the mechanisms at its core.

As well as being the bedrock of all mental phenomena, unconscious phantasy is the primary content of the baby's mind. As soon as the baby is born, he is under the sway of powerful instincts and at the same time he has to deal with the impact of reality on the gratification of such instincts (Segal, 1988). In keeping with object-relations theory, Klein believes that instincts are always represented in unconscious phantasy as linked with the objects at which they aim for their satisfaction. For the newly born baby the first object is typified by the mother or, rather, by the mother's breast. As Klein (1936: 290–291) explains:

> the tiny child is only concerned with his immediate gratification or the lack of it; Freud called this the 'pleasure-pain principle'. Thus the breast of the mother which gives gratification or denies it becomes, in the mind of the child, imbued with the characteristics of good and evil.

The baby desires the breast and perceives it as the source of goodness through the gratification of a good feed. At the same time he will experience frustration from the breast, when left to scream in hunger by the absence of it. However, the undeveloped psyche of the infant is not capable of comprehending absence, and hence construes it as badness. Hence the two opposing aspects of the breast will form separate phantasies of two breasts, one which gives milk, pleasure and love to the baby (the so called 'good breast') and one which withholds milk, causes pain and ultimately is perceived as hateful towards the baby (the so called 'bad breast'). The infant's mind relates to the split breasts by projection and introjection (Klein, 1946: 2), the fundamental psychic mechanisms underpinning unconscious phantasy.

Projection and introjection

In unconscious phantasy, the goodness attributed to the good breast is a mixture of the child's loving feelings for it (part of his Eros) and the experience of satisfaction coming from the real feed; conversely the badness attributed to the bad breast is a mixture of the child's aggressive feelings (part of his death instinct) and the experience of frustration. The wish for the baby to have goodness inside himself will result in the good breast being introjected (i.e. perceived as inside) by the infant's mind so that he can take the goodness inside him to warrant it always being available and secure. At the same time, in response to the threat of annihilation posed by the bad breast, the infant's mind will project the bad breast into the actual breast (the mother's breast), perceiving it as outside of itself.

Freud had anticipated the existence of the mechanisms of projection and introjection as operations that influence the development of the ego. In a description of how the primitive ego conceives the instincts and their objects, his view comes to be strikingly similar to that of Melanie Klein:

> Expressed in the language of the oldest – the oral – instinctual impulses, the judgment is: 'I should like to eat this', or 'I should like to spit it out'; and, put more generally: 'I should like to take this into myself and to keep that out.' That is to say: 'It shall be inside me' or 'it shall be outside me'. As I have shown elsewhere, the original pleasure-ego wants to introject into itself everything that is good and to eject from itself everything that is bad. What is bad, what is alien to the ego and what is external are, to begin with, identical.
>
> (Freud, 1925b: 237)

According to Klein's theory, and resonating with Freud's own suppositions, the basic function of introjection and projection is to allow the baby's ego to free itself from its own aggressiveness, corresponding to its death instinct, and retain the goodness derived from the life instinct inside. However the state of things is not so simple. Because the mother's breast has been imbued with badness and hostility by projection of the bad breast, the baby feels that the mother's breast has become threatening, capable of attacking him and giving him a sense of persecution. Hence, at times when the baby is under the influence of such powerful persecutory feelings, his psyche will project the good breast into the mother's breast with the aim of placing it outside, where it may be kept safer. Equally, the bad breast, which is apprehended as a persecutor, may be introjected, taken inside, as a way of gaining control over it, although this introjection makes the baby feel bad himself.

These movements of objects outside and inside the baby's psyche are continuous: the newborn infant, who has become an individuated body through the rupture of the fusion with his mother and the expulsion from her body, now confronts the task of becoming an individuated mind. To use a bodily metaphor, it is like the baby's mind has retained after birth an umbilical cord attached to his mother's mind, through which 'objects' move in and out, to and fro, and are gradually used to build the baby's own individuated mind. As Kristeva (2001: 62–63) elucidates: 'the fragile ego is not truly separated in the sense of a "subject" separated from an "object", but it incessantly consumes the breast from within and ejects the breast into the outside world by constructing-vacating itself while constructing-vacating the Other'.

In her paper *On identification* Klein (1955: 141) explains that 'introjection and projection operate from the beginning of post-natal life and constantly interact. This interaction both builds up the internal world and shapes the picture of external reality'. Through the processes of projection and introjection, in unconscious phantasy objects become the basis of identification between the baby and the mother.

> In these various phantasies, the ego takes possession by projection of an external object – first of all the mother – and makes it into an extension of the self. The object becomes to some extent a representative of the ego, and these processes are in my view the basis for identification by projection or 'projective identification'. Identification by introjection and identification by projection appear to be complementary processes.
>
> (Klein, 1952b: 68–69)

Identificatory mechanisms start in the infant's psyche in relation to the breast, but continue throughout life, first in relation to the mother and gradually to the father and other people (Klein, 1936). Her clinical experience convinced Klein (1955: 155) that patterns of introjection and projection comparable to those of infancy continue to operate in the adult mind; as she puts it: 'the external world is again and again taken in and put out – re-introjected and re-projected'. Object-relations theory places unconscious phantasy, and the mechanisms of projection and introjection underpinning it, at the core of all psychic phenomena, even when this is not apparent, as is the case in most adult psychic activity. According to Klein and her collaborators, unconscious phantasy constitutes the basis of all psychic development and the foundation of any psychic function (Riviere, 1989). This is most evident in the baby and the young child, where other more sophisticated psychic processes such as language, rationality and critical judgement have not yet developed. Nonetheless the mechanisms of unconscious phantasy are absolutely relevant to the adult, because they 'exert a continuous and powerful influence on the emotional and intellectual life of the individual' (Klein, 1936: 290). Paradigmatically, unconscious phantasy gets expressed in the transference, and projection and introjection are the mechanisms underpinning its unconscious re-enactments (Klein, 1952a). The analyst has therefore a privileged viewpoint into unconscious phantasy and its functioning in the adult's mind through transference.

Ego-splitting and integration

The psychic situation in which projection and introjection take place is a peculiar one, because the binding between the instincts generating from the baby's id and the objects of the external world is so tight that the primitive ego needs to lose a part of itself whenever he projects the object outside. This means that the splitting of the object into good and bad (the good and the bad breast) corresponds to a parallel splitting of the ego (Klein, 1946), whereby the aggressive impulses follow the fate of the bad object (whether this is projected or re-introjected) and the life instincts move in and out of the mind bound with the good object. As Melanie Klein (1946: 6) explains:

> I believe that the ego is incapable of splitting the object – internal and external – without a corresponding splitting taking place within the ego. Therefore the phantasies and feelings about the state of the internal object vitally influence the structure of the ego. [. . .] It is in phantasy that the infant splits the object and the self, but the effect of this phantasy is a very real one [. . .].

Freud (1923: 31) had also noticed the phenomenon of ego-splitting and had presumed the possibility that identificatory mechanisms could result in 'conflicts between the various identifications into which the ego comes apart, conflicts that cannot after all be described as entirely pathological'. Freud had therefore adumbrated the possibility that split-off parts of the ego may exist side-by-side, causing internal conflict, even in healthy minds. These split-off parts remain as unconscious mental objects and get expressed in repetition-compulsion, forming the basis for transference re-enactments.

Although the mechanism of splitting is predominant in the first few months of life, due to the fragility of the infantile ego and its as yet scant ability to deal with external reality, the introjection of the good object and the tendency of the life instinct to promote integration concur in the development of the ego: 'This first internal good object acts as a focal point in the ego. It counteracts the processes of splitting and dispersal, makes for cohesiveness and integration, and is instrumental in building up the ego' (Klein, 1946: 6). Klein devises her own terminology to describe this shift. She names the psychic situation in which the ego is dominated by splitting, the paranoid-schizoid position (Klein, 1952b). The term indicates both that the fragile ego is split in phantasy (schizoid) and also that within this split, the ego feels at the mercy of the perils posed by the bad object (paranoid), because the bad object is either felt to be threatening it from the outside, or filling it with badness from the inside. It is the inability of the baby's mind to comprehend absence that created the phantasy of the bad object: the frustrated instinct cannot be conceived to have been left without an object because that feeling would imply the appraisal of a separation between the object and the baby's self. Hence the frustrated instinct coupled with the absent object is construed in phantasy as a bad object.

The introjection of the good breast enhances the ego's potential to tolerate frustration and perceive the absence of the object. This psychic state is defined by Klein (1952b) as the depressive position.[3] In the depressive position, the perception of absence allows the baby's mind to understand that the good and bad breasts are indeed one and the same. The bad breast is nothing else but the absent good breast. Klein believes that this recognition makes the baby sad (hence the name depressive position) because he realizes that his aggressive impulses have been directed towards the one and the same breast that he also loved. He now feels less persecuted by the object, because the all-bad breast does not exist as such, but he has also lost the idealized all-good breast. He is left with a more realistic object, a 'good enough' mother (to use Winnicott's (1953) phrase) who can satisfy his needs but can also at times frustrate them by being absent. This new psychic state promotes ego development: the integration of the object promotes the integration of the ego. This in turn increases the ego's capability of perceiving external reality, what in Freud's terms would correspond to the predominance of the reality principle. Finally, the increased capacity of the integrated ego for perceiving reality establishes its ability to distinguish between self and 'other' (Klein, 1946). The phenomenon of integration is a progressive one and the baby moves from a relationship to the breast to the perception of the mother as a person, and, gradually, of the father and other people around him: 'Out of the alternating processes of disintegration and integration develops gradually a more integrated ego. [. . .] The infant's relation to parts of his mother's body, focusing on her breast, gradually changes into a relation to her as a person' (Klein, 1952b: 71).

The birth of the self

Ultimately the distinction between the paranoid-schizoid position and the depressive position resides in the fact that only in the depressive position is psychic reality acknowledged as such, and it is because of this recognition that one's own selfhood can be distinguished from that of others. In the paranoid-schizoid position, the inability to understand one's own mind results in the use of the primitive functions of projection and introjection as the basic solution for disencumbering the ego from painful feelings and appropriating an inner sense of pleasure. This however is never definitive, because new frustrations are bound to generate yet more pain and need for projection and introjection. In these cycles the ego becomes split and ultimately pleasure is forestalled. It is only in the depressive position that acknowledgment of the absence of the object will enable the recognition of one's own psychic reality as distinguished from that of the other. But in fact, the depressive position can only come about as a consequence of the paranoid-schizoid one. Repeated cycles of projection and introjection are necessary to establish the dynamic relationship between internal and external reality, before these can be construed as distinct.

While Klein, departing from her work with children, arrives at a description of the beginnings of psychic life intended in developmental terms, her theory, supported by extensive analytic work with adults conducted by her and her collaborators, establishes that the fluctuation between the paranoid-schizoid position and the depressive position is the foundation of all mental activity throughout life. In Klein's (1955: 144) words: 'The tendency towards integration, which is concurrent with splitting, I assume to be, from earliest infancy, a dominant feature of mental life'. Reality-thinking, as the predominant modus operandi of the mature ego and hence of the adult's mind, is grounded in unconscious phantasy (Isaacs, 1989: 109). Moreover, character and personality are indeed based on the work of unconscious phantasy (Isaacs, 1989: 101). Projection and introjection, as processes of unconscious identification which confuse self and other, ultimately lead to the formation of the self, that is, of one's conscious sense of identity.

In the paranoid-schizoid position, the inability of the ego to distinguish between internal and external reality entails a sense of omnipotence for which the infantile ego believes itself in control of its objects and such control is construed as an action. Because the ego is not aware of the psychic aspect of these operations, it understands them as 'deeds' (Isaacs, 1989: 85). Freud had a similar conception of the most primitive and unconscious mental processes being experienced as actions when he talked of repetition-compulsion as the psychic activity 'beyond the pleasure principle' (Freud, 1920). Translated into Freud's terminology, the paranoid-schizoid position corresponds to the psychic function of repetition-compulsion: unconscious emotions are not available for conscious appraisal, and are instead 'acted out' in phantasy as dramatizations through which the split ego and its objects relate to each other, without ever being framed in relation to the self. Whether the baby experiences a bad breast attacking the good baby, or a bad baby attacking the good breast (in the first case the bad object being projected outside, in the second case introjected), psychic functioning remains at the level of unconscious phantasy and the positions of objects inside or outside of the baby are constantly swapped. The perception of outside or inside does not correspond to the awareness of a self as distinct from the other. In the depressive position, instead, psychic functioning operates through the ability to comprehend absence and within recognition of a differentiation between self and other, which enables the apprehension of one's own psychic reality. Although Freud could not have expressed it in these terms, it could be said that the transition between transference re-enactment and transference analysis amounts to a transition of psychic functioning between the paranoid-schizoid position and the depressive position.

As we have seen, the promotion of self-awareness through transference analysis depends on the attitude that the analyst takes towards the patient's re-enactments. Melanie Klein's notion that it is the introjection of the good object which facilitates the transition to the depressive position hints at the role of the mother, given that the good object partly depends on the satisfactions of the baby's needs that the mother grants him. However, it will be left to Bion to expand on Klein's theory and to elucidate the mechanisms by which the mother's mind promotes psychic development in the baby. Or, to put it another way, while Klein focused on the development of the self and the mental operations that support it, Bion will extend the enquiry into that psychic process in the 'other' which is instrumental for the development of the self. This he will call an alpha-function, as we shall consider next.

Bion's theory of alpha-function

Like Klein, and being himself part of her circle in the first part of his career as psychoanalyst, Bion (1984a: 25) starts from Freud's idea that the ego develops from the id with 'the function of establishing contact between psychic and external reality'. Still occupying himself with the unconscious processes that contribute to the development of the ego, he extends the enquiry from the mechanisms inside the baby's mind (unconscious phantasy and the intrinsic mechanisms of projection and introjection) to the occurrences in the mother's mind. These must be essential to the development of the baby's ego, if it is true that the mind of the baby grows not independently of what happens outside of it, but in a mutual and continuous interaction with the mind of the mother, and indeed of that of other people who take care of him. Melanie Klein had moved the focus of enquiry from the relationship between the id and the ego, to the relationship between the ego and its objects. Her description focused on the vicissitudes of the objects in the baby's mind, such as the introjection and projection of the good and bad breast in unconscious phantasy. While she acknowledged the importance of external factors in determining the development of the ego and the shift between the paranoid-schizoid and the depressive position, she did not describe the processes in the mother's mind which promote or hinder this development.

Projective identification

Bion takes a particular interest in identification by projection, or 'projective identification'. Melanie Klein (1946: 8) had used this term to emphasize the fact that projection not only allows the ego to get rid of painful or unwanted objects, but also results in a sense of identification with the object into which the projection is effected. However, she restricted the experience of identification to the child's unconscious and did not explore whether the projection would also induce a sense of identification in the mother herself. Bion, instead, reads projective identification not just as a psychic act of representation – the child or the subject representing to himself the evacuation of an internal object in unconscious phantasy – but also as an act of communication through which the projection effectively speaks to the other person's unconscious. Bion (1984b: 146) maintains that:

> There is a field of emotional force in which the individuals seem to lose their boundaries as individuals and become 'areas' around and through which emotions play at will. Psycho-analyst and patient cannot exempt themselves from the emotional field.

Projective identification is in effect an unconscious communication between two minds, a phenomenon whose existence Freud had envisaged. In a paper aimed at instructing physicians on the technique of psychoanalysis, he gave the following advice to the analyst: that 'he must turn his own unconscious like a receptive organ towards the transmitting unconscious of the patient' (Freud, 1912: 115). Bion (1984a: 90) rendered this meaning with a pictorial image when he designated the recipient of the projection, the mother's or analyst's mind, with the word 'container' and the projection itself with the word 'contained'.

Projective identification is recognized as having a great bearing on what goes on during a psychoanalytic session, representing the way in which the analyst can understand her patients' unconscious communication, beyond the words that they speak. The projection of the objects into another person (specifically the mother in the case of the baby, or the analyst in the case of the patient), is for Bion (1984b) a communicative experience: projective identification is a communication to the mother of unmanageable feelings in the hope that she will experience them, understand them and give them back in a manageable form. Therefore, according to this model, not only the recipient of the projection feels what is projected into her, but also she can act on the projection and transform it, through what Bion will call an alpha-function. Reading Bion's theoretical system through Klein's terminology, it could be argued that unconscious phantasy is the realm of unconscious communication and meaning-making, actualized through projective identification and alpha-function.

Alpha-function

In order to understand what Bion means by alpha-function, it is useful to explain his theory of thinking and the specific terminology he employs. According to Bion, the primitive form of experiencing an emotion is of a thing-in-itself (the bad or good object in Kleinian terms). This mode of psychic functioning is what Melanie Klein described for the paranoid-schizoid position: the baby experiences the distress caused by the absence of the breast when he needs it for comfort or feeding, as a bad breast, a concrete object, a thing-in-itself. It is only with the shift to the depressive position that the baby, learning to understand absence, can integrate the split parts of the object and apprehend the difference between self and other. Filling the gaps in understanding left by Klein's theory, Bion proposed that the transition between the paranoid-schizoid position and the depressive position is characterized by the development of a thinking apparatus that can transform things-in-themselves into thoughts.

Bion postulates that things-in-themselves are 'thoughts without a thinker' (Symington and Symington, 1996: 102) and 'thinking has to be developed as a method or apparatus for dealing with "thoughts" ' (Bion, 1984a: 83). Things-in-themselves are primitive forms of emotional experience that lack a thinker, because the ego has not yet developed the capability of thinking about them. 'Thoughts without a thinker' are only fit for projective identification and are called by Bion (1984a: 6) 'beta-elements'. It is because beta-elements (or things-in themselves, thoughts without a thinker, concrete objects, whichever we choose to call them) cannot be thought about, that they are only

> suited for use in projective identification. They are influential in producing acting out. They are objects that can be evacuated or used for a kind of thinking that depends on manipulation of what are felt to be things in themselves as if to substitute such manipulation for words or ideas.
>
> (Bion, 1984a: 6)

By placing beta-elements into the mother, the baby is not only getting rid of them from his own mind, but also communicating them so that they can be transformed into thoughts. As Bion (1984b: 106) explains: 'Projective identification makes it possible for him to investigate his own feelings in a personality powerful enough to contain them'.

The beta-element placed in the mother's mind is transformed, through alpha-function, into an alpha-element, which can then be returned to the baby as a thought. According to Bion (1984a: 8):

> alpha-function must operate on the awareness of the emotional experience; alpha-elements are produced from the impressions of the experience; these are thus made storable and available for dream thoughts and for unconscious waking thinking. [. . .] Alpha-function is needed for conscious thinking and reasoning and for the relegation of thinking to the unconscious when it is necessary to disencumber consciousness of the burden of thought.

Once the beta-elements are processed through alpha-function and are transformed into alpha-elements, they become available within the ego, where they can be used in conscious thought, or they can be stored as preconscious elements; their new nature does not make them conscious at all times, but easily available for conscious thought when needed, as it is the case for preconscious ideas.

The transformation of beta-elements into alpha-elements is essential for psychic development as much as food and drink are essential for physical growth:

> A central part is played by alpha-function in transforming an emotional experience into alpha-elements because a sense of reality matters to the individual in the way that food, drink, air and excretion of waste products matter. Failure to eat, drink or breathe properly has disastrous consequences for life itself. Failure to use the emotional experience produces a comparable disaster in the development of the personality.
>
> (Bion, 1984a: 42)

By the re-introjection of alpha-elements, which have been produced in the mother's mind by the transformation of the baby's beta-elements, the infant's psyche can develop the capacity for thinking. Its emotional experience is no longer a concrete, unthinkable 'thing-in-itself' but rather a thought, an abstraction that has given meaning to the emotion. 'Alpha function endows the mind with a sense of subjectivity. Now the mind can think about itself and have a personal response to emotional occurrences. It is able to transform the basic emotional experience into thought' (Symington and Symington, 1996: 63).

Because the newborn baby has hardly any capacity for alpha-function, his mother's alpha-function will be crucial for his psychic survival. However, repeated cycles of introjection of alpha-elements will trigger the development of the baby's autonomous alpha-function, which he can then gradually apply to his own emotional experiences, becoming partly independent from the mother. Through projective identification,

> the infant communicates his emotional state to his mother. Her ability to tolerate and process these feeling states, especially the frightening ones, enables the infant to take them back in a manageable form and also gradually to introject this capacity to process emotional experiences.
>
> (Symington and Symington, 1996: 154)

The development of the baby's autonomous alpha-function probably underpins the value of play. As brought to notice by Klein and her circle, from the first few weeks of life, 'the infant spends an increasing amount of time in experimentative play, which is, at one and the same time, an attempt to adapt to reality and an active means of expressing phantasy' (Isaacs, 1989: 97–98). By projecting his objects into the external world, like Freud's grandson did with the cotton reel, the child experiments with unconscious identifications in phantasy. His own alpha-function is then set in motion in relation to the raw emotional experiences represented by the objects, and used to produce meaning. According to Bion's theory, this would only be possible inasmuch as the child has already introjected alpha-elements in relation to this particular emotional situation (for instance, in the case of Freud's grandson, the situation of being left by the mother) and hence has developed at least a rudimentary ability for autonomous alpha-function. Freud's grandson might have experienced previous partings from the mother, when as a baby she left him in his cot, and her returning to soothe him might have provided the alpha-elements necessary for the processing of later emotional experiences of similar kind.

The work with patients in psychoanalysis shows two important aspects of alpha-function. On the one hand, cases when alpha-function hardly develops at all are rare, and present themselves as serious psychotic illnesses in which emotional experiences are not understood and remain as things-in-themselves that haunt the patient in the forms of delusions and hallucinations. On the other hand, neurotic patients and even healthy people have areas of their personality which remain 'psychotic', or split off from the integrated ego. These areas harbour beta-elements for which an internal capacity for autonomous alpha-function has not developed (although autonomous alpha-function may be well developed with regards many other forms of emotional experience). These beta-elements are then expressed as re-enactments and become evident as such in the transference. Anyone, including the mother, or indeed the analyst, had a need as a baby for other people to perform alpha-function on their behalf; moreover, even in their maturity, anyone is most likely to harbour beta-elements in their psychotic area of the personality, where alpha-function is inoperative. Because alpha-function is established and promoted through the 'other', its transpersonal aspect is crucial. That explains why psychoanalysts need to undergo their own analysis for many years during their training, and they tend to return to analysis as patients, from time to time, during their working life.

The double nature of alpha-function

Alpha-function is the capacity to apply one's own understanding to an emotional experience: 'An understanding mother is able to experience the feeling of dread, that this baby was striving to deal with by projective identification, and yet retain a balanced outlook' (Bion, 1984b: 104). In order to be subjected to alpha-function, the beta-element, in projective identification, must be experienced by the mother as if it were her own feeling. When the baby projects the bad breast into the mother, the mother feels the distress of the baby as if it was hers; in fact in projective identification she has 'become' it. Bion distinguishes between a situation when a psychic reality corresponding to a beta-element is inferred and a situation when it is intuited. If the mother knows that the baby is in distress because she sees him crying and hears his screams, this is very different from a situation when the mother intuits the baby's distress because she becomes it. Only in this second case can alpha-function be put into effect, because it is provided with the raw material necessary for its operation.

The emotional understanding that alpha-function fosters is therefore of a very special kind, and should not be confused with a rational appraisal of a situation. As explained by two eminent psychoanalysts:

> The case where you see someone blushing and infer shame is quite different to the one where the analyst *intuits* shame. In the one case it is outside and in

> the other the analyst has *become* it. A psychic reality is only known by being 'become' first. What we have said of shame goes for grief, joy, envy, love, hatred, gratitude, meanness, anxiety and all the emotions.
>
> (Symington and Symington, 1996: 167)

In operating alpha-function, the mother (or the analyst) has to become the emotional experience in order to abstract it into a thought and make it available for emotional development. In this sense, alpha-function can be described as having a double nature, one of feeling and one of thinking, which are not in opposition to each other and do not represent alternative modalities. On the contrary, the emotional experience and the understanding of it are in a reciprocal dynamic relationship: one could not exist without the other. The theory of alpha-function posits therefore a particular form of connection between feeling and thinking: in developmental terms, thinking emerges from feeling, and therefore all psychic functions are ultimately grounded in feeling. This notion evokes the philosophy of the mind advanced by the eighteenth-century theory of sensism. Significantly though, the generation of thinking out of feeling is only possible by the interposition of alpha-function, in itself a form of thinking; this 'chicken-egg' situation postulates a necessary transpersonal dimension of psychic development whereby psychic development is not an insulated activity that happens within the individual mind, but rather depends upon the operations of the more evolved mind of another. As we shall see in the next chapter, the complex nature of alpha-function, with its primary role in psychic development and its transpersonal quality, will prove a reliable framework to understand unconscious emotional processing in acting and spectating.

Notes

1 Freud, writing in German, called these three agencies, Es, Ich and Über-Ich, whose exact English translation would have been 'It, I, Over-I'.
2 In psychoanalytic terms 'cathexis' means the investment of libidinal energy onto an object, for instance the desire for the breast that the baby experiences as part of its instinctual constitution, or the desire for the mother's love which is a prototype for all future loving relationships.
3 The depressive position (psychic state) should not be confused with depression (clinical disorder); in psychoanalytic terms, depression is considered a defence against transition into the depressive position.

Bibliography

Bion, W. R. (1984a) *Learning from Experience*, London: Karnac.
Bion, W. R. (1984b) *Second Thoughts*, London: Karnac.
Freud, S. (1900) 'The Interpretation of Dreams', *The Standard Edition of the Complete Psychological Works of Sigmund Freud, Volume IV and V (1900)*, pp. ix–627, London: The Hogarth Press.
Freud, S. (1909) 'Analysis of a Phobia in a Five-Year-Old Boy', *The Standard Edition of the Complete Psychological Works of Sigmund Freud, Volume X (1909): Two Case Histories: "Little Hans" and the "Rat Man"*, pp. 1–150, London: The Hogarth Press.

Freud, S. (1912) 'Recommendations to Physicians Practising Psycho-Analysis', *The Standard Edition of the Complete Psychological Works of Sigmund Freud, Volume XII (1911–1913): The Case of Schreber, Papers on Technique and Other Works*, pp. 109–120, London: The Hogarth Press.

Freud, S. (1915a) 'Instincts and Their Vicissitudes', *The Standard Edition of the Complete Psychological Works of Sigmund Freud, Volume XIV (1914–1916): On the History of the Psycho-Analytic Movement, Papers on Metapsychology and Other Works*, pp. 109–140, London: The Hogarth Press.

Freud, S. (1915b) 'The Unconscious', *The Standard Edition of the Complete Psychological Works of Sigmund Freud, Volume XIV (1914–1916): On the History of the Psycho-Analytic Movement, Papers on Metapsychology and Other Works*, pp. 159–215, London: The Hogarth Press.

Freud, S. (1920) 'Beyond the Pleasure Principle', *The Standard Edition of the Complete Psychological Works of Sigmund Freud, Volume XVIII (1920–1922): Beyond the Pleasure Principle, Group Psychology and Other Works*, pp. 1–64, London: The Hogarth Press.

Freud, S. (1923) 'The Ego and the Id', *The Standard Edition of the Complete Psychological Works of Sigmund Freud, Volume XIX (1923–1925): The Ego and the Id and Other Works*, pp. 1–66, London: The Hogarth Press.

Freud, S. (1924) 'A Short Account of Psycho-Analysis (1924 [1923])', *The Standard Edition of the Complete Psychological Works of Sigmund Freud, Volume XIX (1923–1925): The Ego and the Id and Other Works*, pp. 189–210, London: The Hogarth Press.

Freud, S. (1925a) 'The Resistances to Psycho-Analysis (1925 [1924])', *The Standard Edition of the Complete Psychological Works of Sigmund Freud, Volume XIX (1923–1925): The Ego and the Id and Other Works*, pp. 211–224, London: The Hogarth Press.

Freud, S. (1925b) 'Negation', *The Standard Edition of the Complete Psychological Works of Sigmund Freud, Volume XIX (1923–1925): The Ego and the Id and Other Works*, pp. 233–240, London: The Hogarth Press.

Freud, S. (1933) 'New Introductory Lectures on Psycho-Analysis (1933 [1932])', *The Standard Edition of the Complete Psychological Works of Sigmund Freud, Volume XXII (1932–1936): New Introductory Lectures on Psycho-Analysis and Other Works*, pp. 3–182, London: The Hogarth Press.

Freud, S. (1938) 'An Outline of Psycho-Analysis', *The Standard Edition of the Complete Psychological Works of Sigmund Freud, Volume XXIII (1937–1939): Moses and Monotheism, An Outline of Psycho-Analysis and Other Works*, pp. 139–208, London: The Hogarth Press.

Freud, S. and Breuer, J. (1895) *Studies on Hysteria: The Standard Edition of the Complete Psychological Works of Sigmund Freud, Volume II (1893–1895)*, London: The Hogarth Press.

Grosskurth, P. (1995) *Melanie Klein: Her World and Her Work*, Northvale, NJ/London: Jason Aronson Inc.

Isaacs, S. (1989) 'The Nature and Function of Phantasy', in *Developments in Psychoanalysis*, edited by M. Klein, P. Heimann, S. Isaacs and J. Riviere, London: Karnac, pp. 67–121.

Klein, M. (1926) 'The Psychological Principles of Early Analysis', in *Love, Guilt and Reparation and Other Works 1921–1945*, London: Vintage, 1998, pp. 128–138.

Klein, M. (1929) 'Personification in the Play of Children', in *Love, Guilt and Reparation and Other Works 1921–1945*, London: Vintage, 1998, pp. 199–209.

Klein, M. (1936) 'Weaning', in *Love, Guilt and Reparation and Other Works 1921–1945*, London: Vintage, 1998, pp. 290–305.

Klein, M. (1946) 'Notes on Some Schizoid Mechanisms', in *Envy and Gratitude and Other Works 1946–1963*, London: Vintage, 1997, pp. 1–24.

Klein, M. (1952a) 'The Origins of Transference', in *Envy and Gratitude and Other Works 1946–1963*, London: Vintage, 1997, pp. 48–56.

Klein, M. (1952b) 'Some Theoretical Conclusions Regarding the Emotional Life of the Infant', in *Envy and Gratitude and Other Works 1946–1963*, London: Vintage, 1997, pp. 61–93.

Klein, M. (1955) 'On Identification', in *Envy and Gratitude and Other Works 1946–1963*, London: Vintage, 1997, pp. 141–175.

Klein, M. (1997) *The Psycho-Analysis of Children*, London: Vintage.

Kristeva, J. (2001) *Melanie Klein*, translated by R. Guberman, New York: Columbia University Press.

McConachie, B. (2008) *Engaging Audiences: A Cognitive Approach to Spectating in the Theatre*, New York: Palgrave Macmillan.

Plato (1986) *Plato: Phaedrus*, translation and commentary by C.J. Rowe, Warminster: Aris and Phillips.

Quinodoz, J.-M. (2005) *Reading Freud: A Chronological Exploration of Freud's Writings*, translated by D. Alcorn, London: Routledge.

Riviere, J. (1989) 'General Introduction', in *Developments in Psychoanalysis*, edited by M. Klein, P. Heimann, S. Isaacs and J. Riviere, London: Karnac, pp. 1–36.

Segal, H. (1988) *Introduction to the Work of Melanie Klein*, London: Karnac.

Segal, H. (1989) *Klein*, London: Karnac.

Symington, J. and Symington, N. (1996) *The Clinical Thinking of Wilfred Bion*, London: Routledge.

Winnicott, D. W. (1953) 'Transitional Objects and Transitional Phenomena – *A Study of the First Not-Me Possession*', *The International Journal of Psycho-Analysis*, vol. 34, pp. 89–97.

Chapter 6

Acting and spectating in alpha-function

The art of the actor as alpha-function

Eighteenth-century theories of acting identified as one of the most contentious issues about the actor's impersonation of her character whether she should feel or not the character's emotions. The mainstay of the rhetorical tradition which had established the continuity between the actor's emotional arousal and the spectator's emotional identification with the character was forever put into question. The subject was discussed in detail and different solutions proposed; the one put forth in Diderot's *Paradoxe* became a paradigm against which future contentions of acting have often been confronted. On the other hand, the so-called emotionalist theory has comparatively been paid little attention, especially in its particulars. In Chapters 3 and 4, I have examined both Diderot's and the emotionalist positions, illustrating the different perspectives from which theorists have understood sensibility, that is, the workings of feelings, in the art of the actor. As I showed, there are especially two features of sensibility which distinguish Diderot's position from the emotionalist one. First of all, there is a difference in what they identify as the object of sensibility: either the actor's own personal feelings, as maintained by Diderot, or rather, according to the emotionalists, the feelings of the character she is called to impersonate. Secondly, their views are also at variance for what concerns the relationship within the actor's mind between her emotional engagement and her study and understanding of the character: for Diderot these are disjointed activities, for the emotionalists they are intrinsically bound to each other. In Chapter 5, I have described in detail how unconscious emotional processing in alpha-function concerns the relationship between unprocessed emotional experiences (beta-elements) and their transformation into emotions endowed with meaning and available to consciousness (alpha-elements). The adoption of a psychoanalytic framework will grant the conceptual and linguistic foundation to solve the conundrum of the question of feeling in the art of the actor.

The relationship between sensibility and understanding in the art of the actor

The psychoanalytic conception of psychic development places unconscious phantasy at the core and origin of all mental activity. Within unconscious phantasy, unconscious emotions are experienced as re-enactments: they are not available to the conscious mind as a thought, but rather lived through as a concrete object-relationship, a kind of dramatic scene. Although unconscious phantasy is especially active in babies and young children, for whom other forms of thinking are just developing, it is also operative in adults, buried within their unconscious mind and harbouring those unprocessed emotions that have been repressed. Repressed emotions are experienced as concrete objects, or beta-elements, which through projective identification give rise to feelings of unconscious emotional identification in which there is no distinction between self and other. They are at the basis of repetition-compulsion, a psychic mechanism which results in compelling re-enactments; these can manifest themselves in everyday life, including as psychiatric symptoms, such as was the case for the Rat Man's obsessions or Anna O.'s hydrophobia. Overcoming repetition-compulsion is possible if the repressed emotions which underpin it are subjected to an alpha-function, a reflective process which gives them meaning and thus brings them into the psychic sphere of the conscious mind, where they contribute to the formation of the self and the development of the personality.

Alpha-function is performed, in psychoanalysis, through the analysis of transference, which is characterized by a dynamic tension between re-enactments and interpretations. During the re-enactment phase of the transference, the patient projects his unprocessed emotions, or beta-elements, into the analyst, who 'becomes' them in projective identification. Such process amounts to an intense emotional experience during which the analyst is unconsciously identified with the patient's emotions and an 'emotional field' (Bion, 1984b: 146) is established between them. The analyst's work of interpretation consists in applying her understanding to the projected emotions: this operation is a function of her judgement, and amounts to giving meaning to the emotional experience, assisted by her knowledge of the patient and of his history. Importantly, though, such understanding is not based on inference or conscious appraisal of a situation, but grounded in her unconscious processing of the emotional experience through her alpha-function. The resulting alpha-elements, namely thoughts pertaining to the emotional experience, can thus be returned to the patient through her interpretation.

The emotionalists identify the true essence of acting in the cooperation between sensibility and judgement, in opposition to Diderot, who describes these two psychic operations as mutually exclusive. It was within the confines of a reflection on the actor which remained overshadowed that sensibility and judgement were postulated to enjoy a complementary and dynamic relationship with each other. As Hill (1755: 54) explains: 'What we should wish in the perfect player is, that he have all the sensibility [. . .] and yet all the command of himself that is necessary to regulate its emotions'. Actors may possess sensibility and understanding in different degrees, and they may employ them in a disjointed fashion, but in these instances they displease the audience; great actors draw upon both qualities so that 'while the judgement regulates the sensibility, the sensibility animates, enlivens, and inspires the understanding' (Hill, 1755: 58). From the perspective of alpha-function, Sainte-Albine's (1749: 2) sibylline remark that under certain conditions '*sentiment* sometimes turns into *esprit*' acquires a clearer meaning. The actor David Garrick (1744: 10) has also given a depiction of acting evocative of alpha-function:

> Wou'd a Player perform [. . .] excellent in *his* Profession, let him be introduc'd into the World, be conversant with *Humours* of every Kind, digest 'em in his *Mind*, let 'em be cherish'd by the *genial Warmth* of his *Conception, transplanted into the fair Garden* of his *Judgment*, there let 'em *ripen to Perfection*, and become *his own.*

The dynamic between sensibility and understanding in the art of the actor can thus be construed as an alpha-function: her becoming the emotions of the character through her sensibility generates an act of understanding. Crucially, such understanding is directed at the character's emotions, not her own, according to a process which is known in theatre jargon as an 'interpretation'. The parallel with what in psychoanalysis is also called an interpretation is conspicuous: the analyst's interpretation happens at the interface between emotional re-enactments and the understanding that the analysis of transference creates. The platform for the analyst's interpretation is the 'emotional field' created by transference. The platform for the actor's interpretation is the character, a fictitious construction. Yet the actor's work of interpretation is aimed at the impersonation of the character in front of an audience. It is therefore the emotional transaction between spectator and actor to which, ultimately, the actor's work of interpretation applies.

The spectator and the transpersonal dimension of acting

According to the emotionalist principle of feeling, which was inherited from classical rhetoric, the actor's emotional arousal is the necessary means to effect the spectator's emotional identification with the character, while the anti-emotionalist position, from François Riccoboni to Diderot, denied that the actor must feel in order for the spectator to feel, but it never came as far as negating the spectator's emotional experience. Instead, Brecht's theory of the *Verfremdungseffekt* demanded the abolition of the emotional identification of both actor and spectator with the character. Notably, whatever opinion theorists chose to hold, they all saw in the transaction between actors and audience the kernel of the spectator's emotional experience.

Brecht's challenge to conventional theatre was grounded in his misgivings about what he saw as the essential ingredients of spectatorship at an emotional level: the passive submission to an emotional identification with the characters, which he defined as 'the empathy operation' (Brecht, 1951: 184). Brecht's terminology tallies with Melanie Klein's definition of empathy as a projective mechanism. According to Klein (1955: 143), who explored most extensively the idea of projective identification in her paper 'On Identification', projective identification is 'the projective mechanism underlying empathy'. What Brecht derogatorily calls 'the empathy operation' entails an unconscious mechanism, or 'hypnotic' to use Brecht's expression, through which the spectator forgets himself and lives vicariously through the character. According to Klein's model of unconscious phantasy, this situation is characteristic of the paranoid-schizoid position, dominated by splitting, projection and introjection. In this psychic constellation, there is a lack of distinction between self and other, because there is no sense of self. Emotions are unprocessed and experienced as concrete object-relations, beta-elements which are only suitable for projective identification.

The immersive emotional identification that spectators experience at the theatre corresponds to the projection of the spectator's beta-elements into the characters. Splitting, which grants the movement of objects inside and outside the mind, enables the co-existence of multiple unconscious emotional identifications effected towards different characters. Thus, although for the sake of simplicity I have spoken generally of projection within a character, projective identification is well suited to effect multiple projections into several characters simultaneously. This psychic mechanism, which was of concern to Brecht for apparently causing the spectator to fall into a hypnotic and submissive state, is of necessity unconscious. This does not mean, as Samuel Johnson (1765: 14) was keen to point out, that the spectator has fallen mad; his mind can retain a sense of reality and the awareness of watching a play, while his unconscious phantasy can at the same time be activated and operate in the paranoid-schizoid position with the projection of beta-elements into the character(s). As pointed out by William Archer (1888: 150) with the theory of dual consciousness, the human mind is capable of working simultaneously on different levels. Therefore, the unconscious operations take place alongside the conscious ones, a condition which makes them more difficult to observe and analyze. In fact, given that they are unconscious, their co-existence with conscious psychic phenomena may justify why their presence could be intuited by so many theorists, but not satisfactorily illustrated.

The projection of the spectator's beta-elements into the character will necessarily be received by the actor who impersonates it. A passage in *The Actor* specifies that sensibility is the 'disposition to receive those impressions by which our own passions are affected' (Hill, 1755: 49), highlighting the function of sensibility as receptacle – or container, to use a psychoanalytic term (Bion, 1984a: 90) – of the emotions. To paraphrase Freud's (1912: 115) advice to the analyst, the actor must turn her unconscious 'like a receptive organ' towards the spectator's unconscious and be ready to receive the spectator's emotions in projective identification. According to the emotionalists, the actor's sensibility is congruous to her fire, intended as her ability to express the character's emotions in such a way that it will arouse the spectator's emotional identification. In other words, the actor's emotional identification is not expressed 'in a vacuum'; there is rather a subtle connection between the actor's expressed emotions and the spectator's emotional arousal, which happens at the level of the impersonation of the character and constitutes, as reported by Archer's respondents, the actor's most powerful means of communicating with the audience. The character's emotions represent the 'emotional field' through which the unconscious emotional communication between actor and spectator is effected.

If she employs the technique advocated by the emotionalists, the actor will steer away from her own personal feelings, so that her own personal emotions will not encumber 'the emotional field'. Like a receptive mother or analyst, the actor's focus on the character's feelings makes her sensibility as soft as wax, available to receive the spectator's projections and to 'become' them in projective identification. Thus, the spectator's projections will provide the raw unconscious emotions on which her work of interpretation can be applied. The projection by the spectator of his beta-elements is the precondition for the activation of transpersonal alpha-function, whose availability will depend, again, on the actor. Through her interpretation, the actor applies her understanding to the character's emotions. Because the spectator has projected his beta-elements into the actor as character, the actor's interpretation will realize the transformation of the spectator's beta-elements into alpha-elements, which will then become available for re-introjection. The introjection of alpha-elements will grant the spectator an emotional awareness in relation to his previously repressed emotions. Through her interpretation, the actor gives meaning to the spectator's repressed emotions, bringing them into his consciousness and promoting the spectator's sense of self.

The art of the actor seen in the light of alpha-function is not an easy labour. It is not an over-statement to compare the actor's dedication to the other, her self-denial, her generosity, to that of the mother for her baby. Her ability to distance herself momentarily from her personal preoccupations, generously putting her mind at the service of the emotions of another, is central to her art. But given its complex nature, alpha-function is not always operative and can be disrupted.

The severing of transpersonal alpha-function

Because of the delicate and complex dynamic between receptive sensibility and emotional understanding that alpha-function entails, the possibility of its failing must be seriously considered. A characteristic situation in psychoanalytic terms is when the projective identification cannot be intuited, and hence the mother (or the analyst) cannot 'become' it. A case in point is that of a depressed mother, whose internal state of self-preoccupation makes her impermeable to the emotions that reach her through a projection. As an attempt to protect her fragile ego, which in depression is usually dominated by the introjection of a bad object, the depressed mother makes herself impermeable to her infant's beta-elements, trying to shut down her emotional responses and therefore obliterating her capacity for alpha-function. Because she maintains enough sense of reality, she can still see and hear her baby's signs of emotions; for instance, she may see and hear her infant crying and make inferences as regards the baby's needs. Thus her practical response to the baby may look similar to that of a mother who is emotionally tuned in, for example, picking up the baby or giving him milk. Notwithstanding, her alpha-function will not be operative because she has not 'become' the baby's emotions, and while her baby's physical needs will have been attended to, his psyche will remain starved.

On the other hand, there are situations when the beta-elements projected into the mother do not encounter a capability for alpha-function because the mother herself is projecting her own beta-elements into the baby. The extreme case would be that of a psychotic mother, who is completely engrossed in her unconscious phantasy to the point that she has lost any sense of reality. This mother will not retain any capacity for responding to her baby, not even on the basis of inference from observation. Although this is an extreme situation, even healthy people may have areas of their personality which are filled with beta-elements and which lack a capacity for processing particular forms of emotional experience. We have seen an example in the case of the Rat Man (Freud, 1909): he suffered from symptoms which disturbed certain areas of his life, in particularly in relation to anger, without his overall functioning being impaired. He harboured aggressive fantasies against the people he loved most and was crippled in certain life situations by his sense of guilt. One extreme example of his psychotic functioning was represented by his obsessions, in which he re-enacted a cruel victimization of his father through a sadistic torture. In psychotic areas of the mind, alpha-function is inoperative. A baby projecting his beta-elements into a psychotic domain of his mother's mind – notwithstanding the mother being able to operate alpha-function in other conditions – will not only be left with his own beta-elements unprocessed, but he will in turn be subjected to the projection of the mother's own beta-elements, greatly hindering his capacity for thinking in this emotional area.

The case of the depressed or the psychotic maternal response can apply to psychoanalysts as well. Although analysts are trained to accept the patient's projections and to maintain a balanced outlook, they always need to be alert for times when they may become impermeable to the projections of their patients' beta-elements or for times when they may be tempted to 'act in'. As we saw in Chapter 2, these are the detrimental responses that Freud (1915) warns against when talking about the erotic transference: either inviting the patient to repress her erotic longings for the analyst, or giving in to the temptation of satisfying them. In order to bring the transference cure to good effect – or, in Bion's terms, to perform her alpha-function for the patient – the analyst is to experience the repressed emotions within her unconscious mind and to interpret their meaning in the context of the transference and the past history of the patient. When this does not happen, the aim of analysis will remain unfulfilled: as Bion (1984a: 6) writes, 'If alpha-function is disturbed, and therefore inoperative, the sense impressions of which the patient is aware and the emotions which he is experiencing remain unchanged'.

As the emotionalists have aptly described, there are situations when actors displease, either because they play their feelings instead of those of the character, or because they feign the character's emotions instead of truly experiencing them. Situations in which actors express their own personal feelings are caused by the application of sensibility without judgement. They entail that form of 'playing by instinct' unanimously deprecated by all eighteenth-century theorists. The actor who plays by instinct, or, to put it another way, who plays her own feelings, is like a mother who responds to the baby's beta-elements with the psychotic part of her personality, or like an analyst who responds to the patient's re-enactments by 'acting in'. Because playing by instinct equates to the withholding of understanding, the actor will not be in a position to transform the spectator's beta-elements through her alpha-function and will return them as unprocessed emotional experiences. Moreover, the actor takes the performance of the character as an opportunity to re-enact her own unprocessed emotions and in turn project her own beta-elements into the audience. Both Diderot and Brecht are similarly concerned about the actor who plays her own feelings, very much along the line of charging her of insanity. In his *Conversation about Being Forced into Empathy*, Brecht (1957c: 270) discusses an anecdote referring to Paulus, an ancient Greek player who has historically come to represent the stock example of an actor who plays her own personal emotions to impersonate a character (Holford-Strevens, 2005). As recounted by Cicero, Paulus was playing Electra mourning the death of her brother. Paulus's son had recently died, and thus the actor took the urn with his ashes on the stage and focusing on his real loss, he shed 'real tears'. According to Cicero the power of the actor's emotional involvement in his own grief made it impossible for the audience to refrain from crying themselves. But Brecht (1957c: 270) is not impressed by this virtuoso performance and comments: 'there is only one word for such an operation: barbaric'. The same anecdote is discussed in the *Paradoxe* alongside the example of the ancient Roman actor Aesopus. While playing King Atreus overtaken by rage, Aesopus hit a servant passing by him on the stage and killed him on the spot (Diderot, 1883: 106–107). Not only does *Premier* suppose both Paulus and Aesopus to be mediocre actors, but he goes as far as calling Aesopus insane and wishing he had been punished with a death sentence: 'He was a madman, and the tribune ought to have sent him straight off to the Tarpeian rock' (Diderot, 1883: 107).

As Hill (1755: 11) lucidly expounds, the extravagance of uncontrolled sensibility not only disgusts the spectator but also induces him to 'despise the player who forces it' upon him. Like a psychotic mother, the actor appears inconsistent, incoherent, extravagant. Like a baby at the hands of a psychotic mother, the spectator will be forced into becoming confused, disgusted, overwhelmed. Brecht's condemnation of the 'empathy operation' acquires meaning when considering that, with actors who play themselves, there is a bilateral movement of beta-elements, not only from the spectator to the actor, but also from the actor to the spectator. The immersive emotional identification to which the spectator yields results in an encumbrance of his unconscious psyche with the beta-elements emanating from the actor's mind. Spectatorship, far from being an opportunity for emotional development, becomes a submission to the actor's unprocessed emotions, which Hill expresses very eloquently when he talks about 'the player who forces it' upon the spectator. Interestingly, Brecht (1957c) will also use the expression 'being forced into empathy' in the title to one of his papers, evocative of the powerful projections that spectators are forced to receive in projective identification when the actor plays her own repressed emotions. Significantly, it is as a solution to the psychotic actor that Diderot and Brecht put forward the concept of the unfeeling actor. Their concern about the emotional damage that a psychotic actor can cause to the audience brings them to champion the option of an actor who keeps her emotional field well apart from that of the spectator's.

According to the emotionalists, the actor who plays by resisting the arousal of feelings within herself is like a deceiving mistress who feigns emotions which she does not feel. While the spectator may be able to tolerate a certain degree of artfulness, ultimately he does not admit that this is in his best interest (Sainte-Albine, 1749: 40). François Riccoboni is an unusual eighteenth-century voice in advocating the lack of the actor's emotional arousal during performance, and the precursor to Diderot's momentous idea of the paradoxical actor. Unlike Brecht, he does not presume that the unfeeling actor will obliterate the spectator's emotional identification with the character; on the contrary, the actor still needs to arouse in the spectator those emotions that she herself does not feel (Riccoboni, 1750: 36). In describing his uneasiness about an actor who feels, he expresses an anxiety that the actor may risk becoming overwhelmed by her emotions:

> If at an emotional point you let yourself be carried away by the feeling of your role, your heart will find itself suddenly shut tight, your voice will be stifled almost completely; if only one tear falls from your eyes, involuntary sobs will hamper your voice box, you will find it impossible to utter one single word without producing ridiculous hiccups.
>
> (Riccoboni, 1750: 37–38)[1]

Similarly to a depressed mother who is unconsciously striving to protect her fragile ego, François Riccoboni's unfeeling actor seems to be engaged in a struggle to deflect the spectator's beta-elements in order to protect her ego from being overwhelmed by projections. The actor who feigns, like a depressed mother, makes herself impermeable to the spectator's projective identifications. A depressed mother may remain competent on a practical level, because inferring the baby's needs from external signs. Her response to the baby may therefore appear indistinguishable from that of a healthy mother. Equally, not all the utterances that the analyst makes during a session derive from her alpha-function, and as such they are not to be considered interpretations in the strict sense of the term. The analyst may provide other forms of response to the patient, some of which may benefit the patient at a conscious level. Patients for instance feel reassured by the analyst's explanation of the causes of a certain symptom. Comments such as 'no wonder that you have problems in controlling your anger given your childhood experiences of aggression at the hands of your father', derived from observation or inference, may improve the patient's conscious understanding of his situation. Notwithstanding, only understandings which derive from an experience of the analyst 'becoming' the patient's unconscious emotions are truly transformative of the unconscious ego, promoting integration and developing subjectivity. Like a depressed mother, or like an analyst who works from inference, an actor who refrains from using her sensibility may appear competent. She can construct an understanding of the character's emotions that may be indistinguishable from the one expressed by a feeling actor. But according to the theory of alpha-function, the experience that she grants the spectator is of a very different kind to that of an actor who can couple understanding with feeling. Because her understanding is based on conscious inference, rather than unconscious intuition, and she has not received the spectator's projective identifications, the spectator's beta-elements will be left untransformed.

Because the actor who acts by instinct can be said, at an unconscious level, to activate the psychotic parts of her personality, I propose to call the style or instances of performing, when an actor plays directly her own emotions, the 'psychotic actor'; on the other hand, I will call the 'depressed actor' the style or instances of an unfeeling actor who makes herself unreceptive to the spectators' projective identifications. My choice of using a terminology whose denotations fall within the language of mental pathology is debatable. I believe that its justification lies in the emphasis I wish to give to the detrimental effect that certain forms of acting may have on the emotional development of the audience. If the availability of the actor's alpha-function is so crucial for fostering the spectator's psychic development, at least for those beta-elements for which he does not possess an autonomous alpha-function, it should not surprise that the art of the actor creates such an aura of controversy.

Diderot's unfeeling actor and the manic position

Diderot's elaboration of François Riccoboni's theory is interesting because with the *Paradoxe* the impossibility of a transaction in feelings between actors and spectators extends into a clear-cut division between spectators who merely feel and actors who merely think. Diderot's paradoxical actor is not, like François Riccoboni's, on the verge of an emotional impossibility; she is indeed deliberately deceitful. It should be specified, however, that Diderot's disparagement for actors' cynical attitude does not seem to extend to those unfeeling actors whom he admires, such as Clairon and Garrick, pointing to another of the many inconsistencies to be found within the *Paradoxe*. Interestingly, it is with specific reference to these esteemed actors that *Premier* hints at the possibility that feeling may have a function in the art of the paradoxical actor. With reference to Clairon, he admits that she may well be engaging her emotions during rehearsals, and that the relinquishing of feeling occurs only at the stage of performance. For what concerns Garrick, he mentions a vague distinction between sensibility and feeling, apparently conceding that feeling may be pertinent to great acting; his remark goes as follows: 'to have sensibility is one thing, to feel [*sentir*] is another. One is a matter of soul, the other of judgement' (Diderot, 1883: 95). These concessions indicate that Diderot had some uncertainties, if feeble, about the principle of the unfeeling actor.

Notwithstanding, returning to *Premier*'s notion of a cynical and unfeeling actor, it is interesting to examine its variation as compared to the depressive style of acting. Departing from Freud's (1917) idea that mania is a mechanism by which the unconscious mind evades depression, Melanie Klein described the manic position as a form of defence against the depressive position. The transition from the paranoid-schizoid position to the depressive position entails ego integration, but it is also characterized by the painful realization that the bad object towards which the baby's aggression was directed is one and the same with the good object. If the ego is too fragile to bear this painful realization, it may either revert back to the paranoid-schizoid position or escape into the manic position. In the paranoid-schizoid position, the ego is trapped in fragmentation and continues to project and introject its split objects, as beta-elements, in unconscious phantasy. In the manic position, the ego employs a '*sense of omnipotence* for the purpose of *controlling and mastering* objects' (Klein, 1935: 277). In unconscious phantasy the ego feels that it is above the influence of objects and it is instead in full control of them:

> This *disparagement of the object's importance and the contempt for it* is, I think, a specific characteristic of mania and enables the ego to effect that partial detachment which we observe side by side with its hunger for objects. Such detachment, which the ego cannot achieve in the depressive position, represents an advance, a fortifying of the ego in relation to its objects.
>
> (Klein, 1935: 163)

Although Melanie Klein does not expand on these points, two aspects of her description are interesting for this discussion. Firstly, the manic position allows the ego to feel in control and fortified with respect to its objects. Its being 'impermeable' to projections is not anymore a strenuous struggle to keep itself from slipping into psychosis, but rather a triumphant sense of being in control and beyond reach of the dangerous effects of the projections. Secondly, in the manic position, the ego is simultaneously 'hungry' for objects, precisely because it believes itself above their power. Likewise, the actors described in the *Paradoxe* are always eager to observe the passions and even the madness of others, by whose effects they remain emotionally untouched. In the passage where he describes actors and other artists as 'the least sensitive of all creatures', *Premier* specifies that they are 'too busy observing, considering, and reproducing' (Diderot, 1883: 13) to be at all touched in their hearts. The manic actor is unaware of her own internal psychic ordeal, much unlike François Riccoboni's depressed actor. Safe in her belief of possessing a superior power of observation and self-mastery, she withholds her alpha-function wilfully in order to let the spectator seethe with his own emotions while she remains detached and controlled. The manic position helpfully explains the nuanced differentiation between François Riccoboni's and Diderot's description of the unfeeling actor, the first endeavouring to shield herself from madness, the second triumphantly delighting in the madness of others. Although both models of actors equally deprive the spectator of transpersonal alpha-function, the actor of the *Paradoxe* adds to her emotional unavailability a malicious ascendancy on the spectator, which risks justifying an outright condemnation of her profession.

The envious spectator

Diderot's notion of the paradoxical actor is not flattering and leads him to describe actors with disparaging words, despite his assertion that he loves and esteems their profession. In the same passage in which he affirms that actors are 'men of a rare talent and a true usefulness, [. . .] the most eloquent preachers of honesty and virtue' (Diderot, 1883: 62), *Premier* insults them with words such as 'caustic', 'cold', 'self-interested', with 'little conduct' and 'no friends', and claims that they are unable to feel compassion: 'I have often seen an actor laugh off the stage; I do not remember to have ever seen one weep' (Diderot, 1883: 63). Diderot's description evokes Rousseau's scathing accusations against the actor in his *Lettre à D'Alembert*, one of the most famous invectives against the theatre of all times. Published in 1758, the *Lettre à D'Alembert* (hereafter cited as *Lettre*) was a response to d'Alembert's article for the VII Volume of the *Encyclopédie*[2] on the Swiss city of Geneva, of which Rousseau was a native. As a city-state, Geneva had an independent statute which banned the performance of plays. In his article, d'Alembert advocated the future establishment of a theatre in the city, adducing its many advantages. D'Alembert argued especially against the supposed immorality of actors, which he presumed to be the main reason behind the proscription of theatre in the city-state. His plea stemmed from the conviction that actors' immoral conduct derived from their marginalization in society, which incited disrespect, prejudice and disdain against them. D'Alembert maintained that if only Geneva could adopt an enlightened attitude towards actors, perhaps compounded by strict laws to regulate their behaviour, it would surely soon be provided with the best acting troupe in Europe and could eventually spread its example to other nations. Rousseau's response was prompt and fierce. Outraged by this public appeal, he took it upon himself to defend his city from the moral debasement that a theatre would threaten to plunge her into. If Plato had wished to ban poets and actors from his ideal city, Rousseau was determined to support the ban already in effect in his city-state.

There are many reasons that Rousseau adduces for his conviction that theatre is at best useless, at worst corrupting. Only some of his considerations are about the moral standing of actors, and they are not flattering. He has no hesitation in proclaiming that the life of actors

> is a state of licentiousness and immorality; that the actors give themselves up to all manner of debauchery; that the actresses lead most scandalous lives; that they are all avaricious, and prodigal at the same time; ever in debt, and

> ever extravagant; heedless in regard to expending their money, and indelicate in regard to the manner of getting it. I find moreover, that in all countries their profession is dishonourable: that they who follow it, excommunicated or not, are every where despised.
>
> (Rousseau, 1759: 97–98)

Rousseau's justification for his critical remarks against actors grounds in the very nature of their art. Rousseau (1759: 103) recognizes as the essence of acting the actor's impersonation of a character that is distinguished from her own person; thus acting is

> the art of counterfeiting, of assuming a strange character, of appearing different from what he really is, of flying into a passion in cold blood, of saying what he does not think as naturally as if he really did think it; in short, of forgetting his own station to personate that of others.

From her ability to play the character, or rather 'every sort of character' (Rousseau, 1759: 103), Rousseau derives the notion that the actor must by necessity be imbibed with the spirit of falsehood. However, pre-emptying possible objections, he needs to concede that the actor is not 'a cheat, who wants to impose upon you' (Rousseau, 1759: 103–104): because the audience know that the actor is feigning, her deceit is inherently harmless. Thus, his condemnation of acting has to take an indirect route: actors are culpable of changing themselves into characters because they do it in order to make money, effectively putting their own person publicly on sale (Rousseau, 1759: 103). Furthermore, their ability to deceive, whilst innocent perhaps at the theatre, becomes the blemish of their personal character:

> Therefore I do not absolutely charge him with being a cheat, but with making it his whole business to cultivate the art of deception, and with practising it in habits, which, though innocent perhaps on the stage, must every where else be subservient to vice.
>
> (Rousseau, 1759: 104)

The censure towards the art of the actor inevitably drifts from a criticism of her art into a denigration of her person. This particular attitude towards actors is interesting because it tallies with yet another mechanism leading to disruption of alpha-function, this time coming from the audience themselves: the situation of the envious spectator.

Bion talks of a particular situation when the mother's alpha-function may be disrupted because of an obstacle in the baby's mind, rather than in the mother's ability to be reflective; this is the case of envy. Melanie Klein (1957) introduced and explored the notion of envy as part of the paranoid-schizoid position. She maintained that the introjection of the good object and the transition into the depressive position, with subsequent integration of the ego, can be hindered by envious impulses. Envy arises from the baby's death instinct and expresses the desire to damage or destroy the good object; envy contrasts with gratitude, which is instead part of the life instinct, and leads to desiring, loving and introjecting the good object. Although the death instinct always plays a part in ego development, envy is particularly prominent in those situations when the death instinct prevails over the life instinct in the baby's psyche. In such instances, integration of the good and bad breasts is hindered and the object remains split into an extreme form of the all-bad breast and the all-good breast. The all-good breast is unrealistically idealized and as such it may be introjected with the projection of the all-bad breast. As Klein (1957: 193) explains: 'Some people deal with their incapacity (derived from excessive envy) to possess a good object by idealizing it'. The idealized object remains as a particularly rigid beta-element and prevents integration of the ego, as its idealization is realized through the juxtaposition with an extremely denigrated object. In the paranoid-schizoid position, the splitting of the object and its precarious status, which subjects it to cycles of projection and introjection, results in the idealized object and the denigrated object easily swapping position from introjection into the ego to their projection, so that the idealized breast (into which the idealized object has been projected) can easily become the disparaged breast.

Bion maintains that when envy prevails in the baby, due to the operations of the death instinct, his projections into the mother have a peculiar quality which disrupts alpha-function. In this case the result of projective identification is felt by the baby to be a further depletion of meaning and a destruction of the thinking process (Symington and Symington, 1996). When this happens in analysis, it may manifest as a resistance on the part of the patient to the analyst's interpretations. The patient is not interested in the analyst's capacity for thinking and alpha-function; on the contrary he wants to destroy it. In this attempt, he may choose to concentrate on asking the analyst questions about her private life, on insinuating that she offers help exclusively because she is interested in the monetary gain, or on dismissing the analyst's attempts at understanding as pointless, stupid or fake. Incidentally, the similarity between such accusations and Rousseau's recriminations against actors is noteworthy. According to Bion (1984a: 91), the relationship between the baby and the mother during alpha-function is 'commensal', because both the baby and the mother gain in psychic growth: 'the mother derives benefit and achieves mental growth from the experience: the infant likewise abstracts benefit and achieves growth'; this explains the engendering of gratitude, which gratifies both baby and mother. On the other hand, an encounter characterized by envy 'precludes a commensal relationship' (Bion, 1984a: 96), and leads to experiencing confusion and meaninglessness.

Following the theory of alpha-function, Rousseau's shift from a criticism of acting into a disparagement of actors can be construed as an unconscious envious attack. Rousseau's misgivings about the possibility of a transpersonal commensal relationship, whereby a shared emotional experience in alpha-function can foster psychic development, drives him to distrust the actor and pre-empt her motives as expedient, exploitative, or at best ungenerous. In psychoanalysis the patient's suspicions that the analyst may just be helping 'for the money', or that she unscrupulously exploits the patient's vulnerability to rejoice in her triumph over him, are powerful defences against the work of analysis. Although it is not impossible that the analyst may be incompetent or corrupted, this is a different situation from when it is the patient's unconscious envy that results in the super-imposition of degrading attributes to the person of the analyst. Radical reading of the theory of alpha-function implies that the deceitful yet competent actor is a phantasy created by the spectator under the impulse of envy. The actor can either be deceitful, in which case she is not competent; or if she is competent, her supposed fraudulence is an unconscious construction on the part of the spectator. It is the ineffectual use of alpha-function that marks the incompetent actor, and this happens when the actor is either psychotic or depressed (with the variant of the manic position). In these instances, her impersonation of the character is ultimately deceitful, as it does not promote the spectator's psychic development. But there are situations when the actor's competence is rendered useless by the disruption of alpha-function through the spectator's envy. In such cases, the deceitfulness of the actor is only apparent: the competent actor is made incompetent in spite of herself.

Brecht's '*Verfremdungseffekt*' and autonomous alpha-function

As human beings, our psychic development is as crucial as our physical one for our survival. Emotions and our ability to make sense of them are the primary nourishment of our minds, which allows them to grow and mature. However, while emotions are, with sensations, the primary content of our psychic experience, we are not born with a thinking apparatus ready to process them and make them available for psychic growth. Such apparatus needs to be established through the caring function of the mother, as much as our other physical needs make us also, as infants, dependent on the mother. As the mother's milk provides the infant with the first necessary nutrients for the development of his body, so the mother's psyche endows him with the rudimentary thoughts necessary for the growth of his mind. Slowly developing a capacity for self-care will eventually make the child virtually independent with regards to his physical needs, although, of course, he will have to rely on the environment, and on social cooperation at various levels, for survival. The introjection of alpha-elements leads, as we have seen, to the development of autonomous alpha-function, making the child, and eventually the adult, capable of processing his own beta-elements. As it was with regards to physical needs, development also grants a growing degree of autonomy with regards to psychic functions, but without ever removing the need for transpersonal emotional processing.[3]

Children use the personifications and impersonations of play to stimulate and develop their autonomous alpha-function. Adults can employ, among other things, works of art. Freud (1908: 144) drew a direct comparison between the playing of children and the creative process of artists:

> The creative writer does the same as the child at play. He creates a world of phantasy which he takes very seriously – that is, which he invests with large amounts of emotion – while separating it sharply from reality. Language has preserved this relationship between children's play and poetic creation. It gives [in German] the name of 'Spiel' ['play'] to those forms of imaginative writing which require to be linked to tangible objects and which are capable of representation. It speaks of a 'Lustspiel' or 'Trauerspiel' ['comedy' or 'tragedy': literally, 'pleasure play' or 'mourning play'] and describes those who carry out the representation as 'Schauspieler' ['players': literally 'show-players'].

Although Freud is specifically talking about the writer and the actor, the reader and the spectator also invest their emotions in the fiction of the book or the play. In doing so, they engage their unconscious phantasy, which can in turn activate their autonomous alpha-function. In this sense it can be argued that all art stimulates unconscious phantasy and fosters autonomous alpha-function. There is an interesting parallel here with the classical definition of *mimēsis*, a complex concept which both Plato and Aristotle employ according to two main connotations: at one level, *mimēsis* pertains to all arts and represents the process at their foundation; at another level, *mimēsis* means dramatic enactment. Moreover, *mimēsis* is an innate propensity, active since childhood, and which facilitates the child's first steps in understanding. In Chapter 2, I have suggested that the arousal of emotions typical of *mimēsis* corresponds to the situation of transference re-enactments, when a patient's unconscious emotions are aroused within the transference, that is to say that *mimēsis* implies the activation of unconscious phantasy. Thus *mimēsis* is characteristic of all arts in as much as they entail the engagement of the audience's (readers', viewers' and so forth) unconscious phantasy and the possibility for autonomous alpha-function. But *mimēsis* also means, more specifically, dramatic enactment, indicating that theatre is a special situation within the arts, amounting to the most primary form of expression of unconscious phantasy and alpha-function: the activation of a transpersonal emotional field, where re-enactments and alpha-function happen across the boundary of self and other.

Given that autonomous alpha-function develops from childhood onwards, and is used in play and in the fruition of art, surely the spectator has some capacity for it to a lesser or greater extent. A theatre performance, like a novel or a painting, or indeed the reading of a play, may provide the framework for the activation of autonomous alpha-function. In this sense, an actor who does not feel the emotions she portrays, while protecting the spectator from the projection of her own beta-elements, still affords an opportunity for the activation of his autonomous alpha-function. This would explain why a 'depressed' actor may be tolerable, while a 'psychotic' one is hardly so: the eighteenth-century emotionalists had been more tolerant, albeit still critical, of the unfeeling actor compared to the psychotic one. If the actor's emotional arousal risks overwhelming the spectator with the actor's beta-elements, it is preferable that the spectator renounces transpersonal alpha-function and relies on his autonomous emotional processing. In explaining his ideas about theatre reception, Brecht (1926: 14) hints at this point: 'The one tribute one can pay the audience is to treat it as thoroughly intelligent. [. . .] The audience has to be a good enough psychologist to make its own sense of the material I put before it'. Reading Brecht's proposition in the light of the theory of alpha-function, it could be argued that while epic theatre obliterates transpersonal alpha-function, the *Verfremdungseffekt* still allows for intra-psychic activation of the spectator's autonomous alpha-function. In other words, the epic theatre does not aim at impeding the spectator's identification with the character, but rather at breaking the unconscious emotional resonance between actor and spectator in projective identification. The character is obliterated in its function of providing the emotional field where actor's and spectator's unconscious minds blend. The distinctive feature of the disruption of transpersonal alpha-function by the *Verfremdungseffekt* is that the actor, while keeping herself impermeable to the projections of the spectator, invites the spectator to adopt an equivalent attitude: both actor and spectator are complicit in exploiting the character as the object of their psychic engagement; neither of them is placed in the vulnerable and reciprocal position of being the object of the projections of the beta-elements of the other.

Although Brecht's model of spectatorship does not distinctly recognize the relevance of productive unconscious processes, still his formulations are evocative of autonomous alpha-function. There is another indication that Brecht's theory of spectatorship may be read as privileging the activation of the spectator's autonomous alpha-function to guard against the risks of projective identification, or empathy: it is his urge for the 'literarization of the theatre' against 'the fact that the theatre can stage anything: it theatres it all down' (Brecht, 1931: 43). Brecht (1931: 44) hopes that through the more literary means employed by the epic theatre, such as the use of titles and film projections, the spectator will be able to adopt a more self-contained attitude, which will empower him to resist the temptation to be 'carried away' in the morass of the transpersonal unconscious.

It is particularly significant that towards the end of his career, Brecht changed his view of the role of empathy in the theatre. By then, he had an extensive experience of the theatre not only as playwright, but crucially, as director. In a series of notes that were written as an appendix to *A Short Organum for the Theatre* and remained unpublished during his lifetime, Brecht (1964: 257) rectified his theory:

> The contradiction between acting (demonstration) and experience (empathy) often leads the uninstructed to suppose that only one or the other can be manifest in the work of the actor [. . .]. In reality we are of course dealing with two mutually hostile processes that are combined in the actor's work [. . .]. The actors derive their true effectiveness from the tussle and tension of the two opposites, and also from their depth.

A long acquaintance with the practice of the theatre seems to have persuaded Brecht that the art of the actor is characterized by the fruitful dynamic between empathy, intended as emotional identification, and acting, intended as the portrayal of the character. As Brecht worked more and more with real actors, it is possible that he became more trusting of their dispositions and also that he better understood the special role that transpersonal identifications play in spectatorship. Perhaps it could be insinuated that alpha-function could not elude his sharp intelligence.

Semiotics and the double game of the actor

In emphasizing the semiotic complexity of a theatrical performance, semioticians have been interested both in constructing systems of analysis which embrace it in its entirety (see for instance Elam, 1980), and also in identifying what may be peculiar about theatre compared to other forms of art. Eco (1977), for instance, highlights that the special semiotic property of theatre is to show, or ostend, real objects as signs. In this aspect, theatre differs from literature, where words are unambiguous artificial signs produced by man in order to communicate (Eco, 1977). It also differs from the visual arts (Helbo, 1985), and even from cinema, in as far as cinema is only a reflection of real presence:

> At the theatre, fiction – it is its force – makes use of real things such as the scenery and the actor, to take form; it then becomes impossible to split what, within the performance, belongs to the one or the other, since theatre performance employs real things to talk about fictional things.
>
> (Pavis, 1985: 73)[4]

Although the property of the theatrical sign to ostend applies to all real objects on stage, including scenery and costumes, the element that is of interest to my discussion pertains specifically to the actor. As theatre semiotics acknowledged from its early days: ‘all that goes on during the performance centers on the actor, so to speak. It is through him that the other components receive their theatrical function and meaning’ (Veltruský, 1981: 230). On stage, the presence of the actor, differently from the words in a literary text or the picture in a painting, ‘has not been actively produced (as one produces a word or draws an image) – it has been *picked up* among the existing physical bodies and it has been shown or *ostended*’ (Eco, 1977: 110). By doing this, theatre leaves open an ambiguity between the body of the actor as natural sign and the body of the actor as artificial sign representing the character. The actor plays ‘a double game: In order to be accepted as a sign, he has to be recognised as a “real” spatio-temporal event, a real human body’ (Eco, 1977: 111). Reading the double game in relation to alpha-function highlights the deep interconnection between embodiment and language which is realized within unconscious emotional processing: while projective identification relies on the person of the actor who needs to be physically present in order to be emotionally receptive, her interpretation is the work of her rational mind which has crystallized within a certain linguistic (intended as symbolic or signifying) rendition of her character; projective identification is always extempore, while the formal aspects of interpretation can be settled, as much as the wording of a poem or the image in a picture. The special skill of the actor is to keep alive the dynamic application of her interpretation to the projections of the audience 'in the moment'; in this sense no performance can be emotionally equal to any other.

In an essay of 1956, Roland Barthes interpreted Brecht's theory of the epic theatre and the *Verfremdungseffekt* as altogether addressing the semiological problem of the double game of the actor: 'For what all Brechtian dramaturgy postulates is that today at least dramatic art should not so much express the real as signify it' (Barthes, 1979: 28). Brecht's (1957b: 154) proposition of the epic actor 'holding himself remote from the character portrayed' is conceived as an attempt at resisting the intrinsic propensity of the theatrical system to conflate the artificial and the natural sign. The tendency of the epic theatre to break the actor's double game in order to magnify its artificial status drives theatre towards renouncing its peculiar quality, which I have identified as the activation of transpersonal alpha-function. If the transpersonal nature of alpha-function is what distinguishes theatre from other non-performative arts, it makes one wonder whether other performing arts such as music, dance and live art also draw upon transpersonal alpha-function; this intriguing question I must leave unanswered.

A further reflection on the double game of the actor affords another interesting insight in relation to the phenomenon of the spectator's envy. As I have contended, the failure of alpha-function can in certain situations be caused by the nature of the spectator's projections, rather than failures in the actor's interpretation. Envy is characterized by extremely split objects, which resist integration: when envy predominates in unconscious phantasy, the projections have a special quality that hinders alpha-function and their transformation into alpha-elements. In analysis, a situation when envy is predominant often manifests itself with an anxiety on the part of the patient to concern himself with the personal life of the analyst, either because of a desire to know her better as a person or with the intent of drawing attention to her shortcomings. Interestingly, disparaging comments against the analyst's professional or personal attitude, praise of her qualities, or concerns about her well-being, as much as they appear disparate, can all be signs of the same envious process, when, unconsciously, they represent the resistance against the function of analysis. This envious attitude reminds, in theatre, of the curiosity that spectators take in actors' private lives. This situation is particularly emphasized by the phenomenon of celebrity actors, a phenomenon which, in semiotic terms, 'splits the acting sign much like the sign is split by Brecht in his *verfremdungseffekt*' (Quinn, 1990: 156) but with opposite results: here the actor is obliterated as artificial sign and magnified as a natural sign; her function is to represent herself. Interestingly, actors often enjoy, in these instances, a form of idealization, which is fragile and unstable and may easily be turned into disparagement. In actual fact, it is typical of envy that: 'The former idealized person is often felt as a persecutor (which shows the origin of idealization as a counterpart to persecution), and into him is projected the subject's envious and critical attitude' (Klein, 1957: 193).

Focussing on the person of the actor outside her function of interpreter of the character may cause spectators to elude the actor's alpha-function. As Quinn (1990: 158) has claimed in his semiotic study of celebrity acting: 'the star's role has the power to overshadow the whole art work'. The spectator's preoccupation with the person of the actor may facilitate an envious engagement of her unconscious phantasy, a resistance against the function of the actor as interpreter of the character and, ultimately, the disruption of alpha-function. If envy impedes alpha-function, it may also be possible that actors who are particularly poor at alpha-function may be especially prone to engendering envy and therefore to becoming idealized or denigrated. Perhaps the reason why the phenomenon of celebrity acting is aggravated by film (Quinn, 1990: 155) is connected with the intrinsic condition that in film actors are exempt from the extempore performance of transpersonal alpha-function on the audience. Whether it is the actor's lack of alpha-function to trigger envy or rather the spectator's envy to disrupt alpha-function remains an open question. If it is true that all real objects resist their use in signification (Quinn, 1990: 155), the art of the actor, which relies precisely on the actor being a real object who simultaneously needs to signify, inevitably harbours a problematic nature.

Unconscious emotional processes of theatre spectatorship

The interest that theorists of the theatre manifest towards the status of spectatorship and of acting can, at least in part, be ascribed to their concerns about the purpose and value of the theatre. Brecht is exemplary: his theoretical preoccupation with the effect of theatre on spectators and the ensuing creation of a new model of acting was strictly tied to his appraisal of the socio-political harm that conventional theatre is supposed to produce. His response was a life-long venture to reform theatre in the direction of making it a tool for political awareness and the amelioration of society. Diderot's project of theatrical renovation was similarly coloured by ethical considerations; his active engagement as playwright and theorist was grounded in his belief that theatre had a role to play in the promotion of moral habits. As has been suggested, 'The [. . .] principal object of Diderot in writing *Le Fils naturel* and in expounding his doctrines was to make the theater an institution for teaching morality' (Wilson, 1972: 270). Diderot's (1939: 149)[5] own claim in the *Entretiens* that the object of drama 'is, I believe, to inspire mankind with love for virtue and horror for vice' is telling. By the time he wrote the *Paradoxe*, Diderot's interest in dramaturgy had become secondary to his radically transformed view of actors. If the fictionalized actors of *Le Fils naturel* were involved in the writing and performing of plays of direct relevance to their immediate social context, the skilful but cynical actors of the *Paradoxe*, far from being vehicles for teaching morality, were now conceived as detached observers of human passions and utterly unconcerned about the amelioration of their fellow men and women. In spite of Diderot's later distrust for actors, both his and Brecht's criticism of the theatre comprised a design to contribute to its reformation. Seen in the light of spectatorship entailing an opportunity for transpersonal alpha-function, their concerns about the effect of theatre on the audience and their dedication to its reform acquire a new significance. In particular it is the role of emotions in mediating the effect of theatre, and the emotional transaction between actor and spectator, which dominates their preoccupations. The same concerns lead detractors of theatre, such as Rousseau, to condemn theatre at all levels without the possibility of appeal.

Theatre for pleasure or theatre for instruction

Rousseau attacks the status of the theatre on its long-standing claim that its aim is to please and instruct. The prototype of this notion comes from Horace, who in his *Ars poetica* (333–334) had written that poetry should either please or instruct, or both: 'Poets aim either to benefit, or to amuse, or to utter words at once both pleasing and helpful to life'. Rousseau highlights what he sees as an absurd contradiction in terms: he accepts that the principal aim of the theatre is to please, because only in this way will the spectators' interest be engaged. But he then turns the implications of this argument upside-down by claiming that spectators will only be pleased by what reinforces their values and beliefs: at best theatre will reinforce already established good habits, at worst it will strengthen existing bad habits (Rousseau, 1759: 17). Therefore, the need for theatre to please is precisely what hinders its potential to morally instruct. In similar terms, the question of pleasure had been an important point of contention between Plato's and Aristotle's evaluations of *mimēsis*. While for Aristotle, the link between *mimēsis* and pleasure is one of the main foundations on which *katharsis*, and hence the desirable effect of tragedy, is based (*Poetics*, 1448b4–1449b28), Plato condemns *mimēsis* and wants to ban it from the ideal city precisely because of its compelling quality intrinsic to the pleasure that it grants (*Republic*, 605c6–8). According to Plato, *mimēsis* promotes in the audience the arousal of feelings that belong to the irrational character to the detriment of reason (*Republic*, 604e1–5). The platonic equivalence between the pleasure of theatre, irrationality and emotional engagement is matched almost word for word by Rousseau. The Genevan philosopher contends that the problem with theatre is precisely that theatre reception is about emotions, not reason. He ridicules the idea that through *katharsis* it may be possible to rescue the mind from the grip that the represented emotions have on spectators:

> I am not ignorant that the poetic art, so far as it regards the theatre, pretends [...] to purge while it excites the passions: but I have great difficulty to understand this rule. Is it that to grow temperate and wise, we should begin with being intemperate and mad?
>
> (Rousseau, 1759: 18)

Like Plato, Rousseau (1759: 19) understands emotional arousal as irrationality, madness even, and sees it as a perilous undercurrent which can amplify itself to a dangerous degree:

> Is it not well known that all the passions are sisters, that one only is sufficient to excite a thousand, and that to combat one by means of another, is the way to render the heart more sensible to them all? The instrument that serves to purge them is reason; and reason [. . .] has no effect upon the stage.

Reason only is capable of overcoming irrational emotionality, but there is no place for reason in the theatre: 'Reason alone is of no use upon the stage. A man without passions, or that has them absolutely under his command, would engage nobody in his favour' (Rousseau, 1759: 15). If there is no place for reason, there is therefore no scope for moral instruction.

The notion that the purpose of the theatre is entertainment and moral improvement has remained a leitmotif across the centuries. The title of one of Brecht's essays, 'Theatre for Pleasure or Theatre for Instruction', epitomizes the problematic nature that he saw in the presumed concurrence of pleasure and instruction in theatre spectatorship. In the essay, Brecht (1957a: 110) explains that the aim of the epic theatre is to break the spectators' empathy with the characters through a process of alienation, so as to shift their attitude from a passive submission to feeling, to an active intellectual curiosity. The dichotomy between empathy and understanding amounts to an antagonism between emotional arousal and rational detachment. As von Held (2011: 21) explains:

> In the age of science and technology, theatre must appeal to the spectator's rational and cognitive rather than emotional interests. Just like a scientist, who with objective distance and cool curiosity observes her research material in order to discover the hidden principles behind it, Brecht wants his spectator to explore sociology through drama.

The insistence on the primacy of reason in mediating theatre's political effect is related to Brecht's particular view of the status of emotional engagement in spectatorship: whether emotions derive from reason or arise independently of it, makes all the difference. This distinction leads Brecht to differentiate between two forms of theatrical pleasure. On one side is the pleasure of empathy, utilized by the Aristotelian theatre to hypnotize the audience and render it acquiescent to the status quo (Brecht, 1930). On the other side, the pleasure afforded by the epic theatre, altogether rejecting empathy, derives from 'the wisdom that comes from the solution of problems, [. . .] the anger that is a practical expression of sympathy with the underdog, [. . .] the respect due to those who respect humanity' (Brecht, 1949: 186). The opposition between empathy and alienation corresponds to the dichotomy between a desirable pleasure derived from instruction and reason, and a harmful pleasure derived from emotions. For Brecht, like it was for Plato and

Rousseau, theatre's harmful effect ensues from the dangerous cocktail of emotional identification and pleasure that spectatorship entails.

Brecht's supposition that instruction needs to generate pleasure for theatre to accomplish its moral purpose is antithetical to Aristotle's conception of the effect of tragedy, where pleasure is thought to engender instruction, an antithesis which should not surprise, given that Brecht's formulation is openly in opposition to that of Aristotle. Aristotle professed that the first aim of poetry (dramatic and non-) is to give pleasure, and moral teaching is at best relegated to be a secondary aim (Butcher, 1951). This is often misapprehended, because Horace's dictum about the moral purpose of poetry was so influential 'that even writers focusing on Aristotle rather than Horace tended to project back onto the theory of catharsis moralistic aims that might appear quite alien to the Greek philosopher' (Harris, 2014: 174). Nevertheless, Aristotle's theory maintains a link between tragedy's aims of aesthetic pleasure and of moral improvement. As a scholar of Aristotle has pointed out:

> The aesthetic representation of character he views under ethical lights, and the different types of character he reduces to moral categories. Still he never allows the moral purpose of the poet or the moral effects of his art to take the place of the artistic end. If the poet fails to produce the proper pleasure, he fails in the specific function of his art. He may be good as a teacher, but as a poet or artist he is bad.
>
> (Butcher, 1951: 238)

This reading of Aristotle suggests that the Greek philosopher did not consider pleasure and moral improvement as mutually exclusive. As Lessing has insightfully indicated, it is possible that Aristotle had an opposite view of the relationship between pleasure and moral improvement to that proposed by Brecht. Giving his own interpretation of Aristotle's theory of tragic *katharsis*, in article 78 of the *Hamburg Dramaturgy*, Lessing (1890: 421) reads *katharsis* as the transformation of pity into virtue: 'whoever has endeavoured to arrive at a just and complete conception of Aristotle's doctrine of the purification of the passions will find that [. . .] this purification rests in nothing else than in the transformation of passions into virtuous habits'. The pleasure implicit in tragic *katharsis* may therefore be construed as the necessary premise to the ethical effect of theatre, in contrast with Brecht's notion that theatrical pleasure inherent to *katharsis* is an obstacle to the ethical function of the theatre.

Perhaps it should puzzle us that Brecht turned his own theory on its head at the end of his career. In a note of 1952, appended to the published version of one of his writings, he declares:

> Recently [. . .] we have given up examining works of art from their poetic (artistic) aspect, and got satisfied from theatrical works that have no sort of poetic appeal and from performances that lack virtuosity. Such works and

> performances may have some effect, but it can hardly be a profound one, not even politically. For it is a peculiarity of the theatrical medium that it communicates awareness and impulses in the form of pleasure: the depth of the awareness and the impulse will correspond to the depth of the pleasure.
>
> (Brecht, 1952: 230)

Here it is not awareness which provokes pleasure, but pleasure which engenders awareness. This shift in Brecht's view comes around the time when he also changes his appraisal of the role of empathy, by recognizing, as we have seen, that a fruitful dynamic between empathy and interpretation is necessary to the art of the actor. Albeit in the passage quoted above Brecht does not intimate that the spectator's pleasure must be connected with empathy, he is explicitly stating that, without inherent pleasure, theatre cannot instigate political change, except for the possibility of a 'shallow' effect.

As is the case with regards to the contention between Aristotle and Plato, the recognition of a link between theatre and pleasure remains throughout history a thorny question. The pleasure implicated in spectatorship can justify the condemnation of theatre (Plato and Rousseau), be taken as a primary effect which is necessary for the ensuing moral effect (Aristotle and the late Brecht), or be thought to be useful insofar as it is generated by an intellectual engagement (Brecht's epic theatre). As indicated by Brecht, the question of pleasure links to the question of emotions, and it is the judgement on the value of emotional identification that ultimately will guide theories about theatre's function.

Theatre spectatorship, emotions and pleasure

The theory of alpha-function distinguishes between two kinds of emotions: beta- and alpha-elements. Beta-elements are primitive forms of emotional experience that lack a thinker, because the ego has not yet developed the capability of thinking about them. Thus they are only fit for projective-identification; through re-enactments, they force themselves on the mind of others and evoke in them unprocessed feelings which, if not subjected to alpha-function, encumber their ego and make them susceptible to 'act in', often resulting in irrational and impulsive responses. It is only when beta-elements are transformed, through alpha-function, into alpha-elements, that they become emotions endowed with meaning, made available for conscious thought. The problematic nature of psychic development lies in the special relationship between feeling and thinking that characterizes emotional processing: unprocessed emotional experiences are, ultimately, the building blocks of our psyche, although in order to be useful for thinking they must be transformed. Alpha-function serves like a metabolic mechanism: from the raw materials of unprocessed emotions it has to extract the useful nutrients of emotions with meaning.

The metabolic function of alpha-function itself, as we have seen, is not available at birth and must be developed from the processing of beta-elements; this makes our psychic development profoundly dependent on the mind of the other. The contention between Plato's and Aristotle's views of *mimēsis* illustrates the conundrum of psychic development. Plato condemns *mimēsis* on the basis of its compelling and irrational quality, as if he was expressing his concern about the activation of unconscious phantasy and the projection of beta-elements that it entails. In point of fact, when beta-elements are projected, they are expressed as re-enactments and, unless they encounter an alpha-function, perpetuate repetition-compulsion, and pose the danger of re-traumatization. On the other hand, when Aristotle grants *mimēsis* the status of necessary foundation for *katharsis*, he seems to recognize that no psychic development would be possible unless rooted in unconscious phantasy and the re-enactments that it entails.

In my interpretation of tragic *katharsis*, I have suggested that *katharsis* may be understood as a transition between a situation of immersive emotional identification (fear) in which the spectator experiences the character's emotions as his own, and a sympathetic detachment (pity) whereby the spectator takes an interest in the character's emotions as compassionate witness. Such transition corresponds to the shift, promoted within the transference, from the unconscious emotional identification of the transference re-enactment, to the self-reflective stance of transference analysis. In this sense, the spectator's transition from fear to pity can be understood as his taking a reflective stance in relation to his own repressed emotions, positing an equivalence between *katharsis* and alpha-function. If the emotional response allowed by *katharsis* amounts to alpha-function, the emotional engagement characteristic of fear corresponds to the activation of an emotional field between spectator and character in projective identification. The emotions in fear would therefore correspond to beta-elements. The transition to pity, instead, would represent the transformation of beta-elements into alpha-elements, sympathetic thoughts which are pertinent to the self. In article 75 of the *Hamburg Dramaturgy*, Lessing gives an interpretation of Aristotelian *katharsis* strikingly similar to the one I propose. He affirms that according to the theory of tragic *katharsis*, fear and pity are not to be aroused in a disjointed way: 'this was not Aristotle's reason; according to his definition of compassion, it of necessity included fear, because nothing could excite our compassion which did not at the same time excite our fear' (Lessing, 1890: 409). Moreover, in article 76 Lessing (1890: 412) specifies that, according to Aristotle, pity is in actual fact best understood as self-referential: 'Compassionate emotions unaccompanied by fear for ourselves, he designates philanthropy, and he only gives the name of compassion to the stronger emotions of this kind which are connected with fear for ourselves'.

The theory of alpha-function affords a particular view of the question of pleasure in spectatorship. In Freudian terms, alpha-function entails the overcoming of repetition-compulsion, which is a psychic mechanism 'beyond the pleasure principle'. The effacement of the compulsive grip that repetition-compulsion has on the mind engenders a sense of agency and the re-establishment of the pleasure and reality principles as the regulators of psychic life. In Kleinian terms, alpha-function promotes the transition to the depressive position, which is characterized by the progressive integration of the ego and of the good and bad object, the abating of persecutory fears, a feeling of greater security, and a drive to make reparation. This transition, which allows for an increased capacity to distinguish the self from the other, marks the insurgence of feelings of gratitude towards the mother (Klein, 1957: 189), now recognized as the caring attendant to the needs of the infant. The pleasure of spectatorship in alpha-function can therefore be said to amount to the pleasure of an enhanced sense of self and to the gratitude that the spectator feels for the actor's gift of alpha-function. Perhaps the sense of obligation for the alpha-elements that actors bestow on the audience underlies the impulse behind the round of applause that rises at the end of a performance and even, at times, during it.

Theatre, empathy and sympathy

It is a cliché that spectatorship entails the bestowing of sympathy on the characters. As I have briefly mentioned in Chapter 1, Rousseau (1759: 24) was very scathing of theatrical sympathy and believed it to be 'a barren pity, fed with a few tears, and never productive of the least act of humanity'. The sympathetic function of spectatorship supposedly corresponds to a shallow participation in a fictional experience that justifies the disavowal of one's own sympathetic duties in real life. Rousseau's example of the bloody Sylla, who cries at the misfortunes of dramatic characters while he continues to do harm to real people in real life, exemplifies this situation. There is however an alternative view of theatrical sympathy, which Diderot put forth in his essay *De la poésie dramatique*. In contradiction of course to his own later views as *Premier*, which are much more akin to those of Rousseau, in *De la poésie dramatique* Diderot (1939: 312) maintained that at a theatrical performance, when wicked men are moved to compassion against the injustices that they themselves commit, this is not a temporary and shallow effect, but a transformative one: 'the impression has been received; it stays with us; and the wicked man exits from his loge less disposed to do harm than if he had been reprimanded by a stern and harsh orator'.[6] Notwithstanding the proliferation of different and contradictory meanings that sympathy (and empathy) has been given both in psychology and literary studies (McCarthy, 1997: 5), alpha-function can provide an original rendition of theatrical sympathy. But in order to discuss sympathy, we also need to return to the formulation of empathy.

As we have seen, empathy is, in Kleinian and Brechtian terms, an accurate designation for the projective mechanisms characteristic of the paranoid-schizoid position. For Klein (1955: 143) projective identification is 'the projective mechanism underlying empathy'. Brecht (1951: 184) identifies the 'empathy operation' as the conflation of the spectator's emotions with those of the character, in a hypnotic experience where the spectator's sense of self is obliterated. For what concerns sympathy, Brecht (1949: 186) mentions it, in opposition to harmful empathy, as a desirable effect of the epic theatre, implying that it facilitates the understanding of the characters' predicament. Klein hints at sympathy as developing out of cycles of projective identification and introjection; transposed into Bion's terminology, sympathy is the outcome of the cycle that, from the projection of beta-elements in projective identification, results in the re-introjection of alpha-elements. Departing from these formulations, and specifically in relation to the unconscious processing of emotions, the emotional identification characteristic of the projection of beta-elements (projective identification) corresponds to empathy, while the sympathetic understanding which results from the re-introjection of alpha-elements (alpha-function) can be named sympathy. According to this model, sympathy is always dependent on empathy, in agreement with Lessing's interpretation of tragic pity as necessarily presupposing fear. This is at variance, as we have seen, with some eighteenth-century definitions of sympathy, in particular Adam Smith's (1976: 9) formulation of the sympathetic imagination, whereby sympathy is grounded in a self-centred experience disjointed from a primary emotional experience of the feelings of others. For Adam Smith empathy as projective identification is not a credible phenomenon, in spite of the fact that its existence had been advanced by his fellow philosopher David Hume. The sympathetic imagination remains grounded in an act of wilful fantasy, rather than in unconscious phantasy, and as such amounts to a solipsistic experience, of little value to the recipient of the sympathy, as well illustrated by Diderot's (1883: 40) encounter with Sedaine.

By extending my proposed designation of empathy and sympathy to Aristotle's theory of tragic *katharsis* and by defining Aristotelian fear as 'empathy' and Aristotelian pity as 'sympathy', we find that Lessing and Klein would concur in ascribing a self-referential nature to sympathy, that is to say that sympathy is first and foremost about an improved understanding of oneself, before it can be applied as a compassionate understanding of another. This point is particularly poignant in relation to theatre spectatorship, because it implies that, through the actor's interpretation, the spectator is sympathized with, challenging the deeply held conviction that in theatre reception the spectator feels sympathy for the character. Interpreting spectatorship as alpha-function instead suggests that, while at a conscious level the spectator may become aware of applying his sympathy to the character, the underpinning unconscious process amounts to the sympathetic response that the actor has bestowed on him. In other words, when the spectator believes that he is sympathizing, he is (also) being sympathized with.

If fear is the necessary root of pity, no act of sympathy can be achieved without previous empathy, and therefore one would have to answer affirmatively to Rousseau's (1759: 18) question: 'Is it that to grow temperate and wise, we should begin with being intemperate and mad?' It is wrong to suppose, like Rousseau does, that empathy with negative characters will inevitably result in the encouragement of vice: if alpha-function is effected, the split-off 'bad objects', used in projective identification with the 'bad characters', will be transformed into thoughts, freeing the mind from the compulsion to repeat and placing the aggressive or destructive impulses under the control of reason. Diderot's rendition of theatrical sympathy in *De la poésie dramatique* illustrates this point.

When Brecht theorized the primacy of reason in the fruition of the epic theatre, he maintained that unconscious emotional arousal was harmful to sympathy, intended as an inferential understanding of the predicament of the characters. The socio-political and ethical function of theatre depended on the conscious imparting of information about social processes. Later in his career, however, he realized that unless theatre took advantage of the fruitful dynamic between empathy and interpretation in the art of the actor, and of the pleasure that this engenders, its potential for socio-political awareness would be obliterated. Perhaps returning to a formulation similar to Aristotle's theory of tragic *katharsis*, he recognized that only an emotional experience grounded in empathy could lead to a transformative process, and that the spectator's emotional engagement and pleasure underlie the ethical function of the theatre.

Semiotics and theatre's feedback loop

Theatre semiotics has emphasized the spectators' active function not only as the recipients of the theatrical communication and the ultimate makers of its meaning, but also as responders. As has been claimed, spectators '*in turn* assume the role of transmitter of signals to the performers [. . .]. This feedback process [. . .] is one of the major distinguishing features of live theatre' (Elam, 1980: 38). Semiotic attempts at defining the actor-audience transaction have had to contend with the difficulty raised by the French linguist George Mounin, who challenged the notion of the actor-spectator relationship as entailing communication, given that there is no sharing of a common communicative code and no reciprocation of roles between sending and receiving messages: in theatre, claims Mounin (1969, cited in Elam, 1980: 33), actors remain the senders and spectators the receivers. This proposition however has been rejected not only by theatre semioticians but also by scholars of other approaches, and, indeed, by actors themselves. For instance, Bennett (1997: 21) recognizes the reciprocal relationship between audience and performance 'even for the most "culinary" theatre' let alone for contemporary theatre events in which the audience is deliberately enticed into a productive role. The Italian actor-playwright Dario Fo (1977: 54–55) talks about the audience response to the actor in terms of laughter, breathing and uneasiness as an instantaneous spur to the actor's own reactions.

While there is hardly any doubt that theatre spectators send live signals during a theatrical performance, the difficulties of semiotics have lain in deciphering the codes of such transaction, and semioticians have resorted to responding to Mounin's challenge by establishing that spectator-actor communication happens through a different set of codes from those of the counter-route of actor-spectator communication (Ruffini, 1974, cited in Elam, 1980: 34). There have also been attempts at discovering a reciprocal code underlying the communicative feedback loop between audience and actors. Notably, in her study of performance with a particular focus on modern forms of participatory theatre, which she sees as testing the nature of the feedback loop, Fischer-Lichte (2008) emphasized the role of embodied perceptions as a powerful communicative code between audience and actors, although she also suggested that this explanation may have limited value for conventional theatre which stages the performance behind the 'fourth wall'. As semiotics has highlighted, the variety of sensory channels involved in theatre spectatorship implies that the 'feedback loop' is effected in multiple ways. Yet alpha-function suggests the existence of a universal channel for the reciprocal communication between actors and audience: the circulation of beta- and alpha-elements through projection and introjection. Such circulation places the spectator in the role of primary emitter, confirming the semiotic contention that spectators are active transmitters of signals. Admittedly, beta-elements are part of a compulsive process, and in this sense their emission could be construed as 'passive', if intended as not under the emitter's control. Notwithstanding, alpha-function challenges the idea of the passive spectator: at an unconscious emotional level theatre spectators are bustling with lively psychic activity. If one considers that the spectators' autonomous alpha-function is also activated by the performance, the image that comes to mind is of an auditorium filled with sparkles of unconscious emotional elements moving across actors' and spectators' minds – not to mention the unconscious emotional transactions at the level of the audience's communal experience; but this is to be left for another conversation.

Notes

1 'Si dans un endroit d'attendrissement vous vous laissez emporter au sentiment de votre rôle, votre cœur se trouvera tout-à-coup serré, votre voix s'étouffera presqu'entierement; s'il tombe une seule larme de vos yeux, des sanglots involontaires vous embarrasseront le gosier, il vous sera impossible de proférer un seul mot sans des hocquets ridicules'.

2 In *Encyclopédie, ou dictionnaire raisonné des sciences, des arts et des métiers, par une société de gens de lettres. Mis en ordre & publié par M. Diderot de l'Académie des Sciences et Belles-Lettres de Prusse, et quant à la partie mathématique, par M. d'Alembert de l'Académie royale des Sciences de Paris, de celle de Prusse et de la Société royale de Londres.* 1751–1772, Vol. 7, p. 578, Paris: Briasson, David, Le Breton, Durand.
Accessed on the web via *The Making of the Modern World.*

3 It is interesting to engage with the observation that the need for social cooperation intrinsic to the survival of the human species may justify, from an evolutionary perspective, why it is advantageous that psychic development remains partly determined by interpersonal dynamics: if human beings are psychologically dependent on each other, they will tend to stick together, even if they could, at least in theory, choose to live in isolation. This will make them stronger as a species. Further analysis of this supposition is outside the remit of my discussion.

4 'Au théâtre, la fiction – c'est là sa force – se sert de choses réelles: la scène, l'acteur, pour prendre forme: il devient alors impossible de scinder ce qui dans la représentation appartient à l'un ou à l'autre, puisque la représentation théâtrale utilise des choses réelles pour parler de choses fictives'.

5 'C'est, je crois, d'inspirer aux hommes l'amour de la vertu, l'horreur du vice'.

6 'l'impression est reçue; elle demeure en nous, malgré nous; et le méchant sort de sa loge, moins disposé à faire le mal, que s'il eût été gourmandé par un orateur sévère et dur'.

Bibliography

Archer, W. (1888) *Masks or Faces: A Study in the Psychology of Acting*, London: Longmans, Green and Company.

Aristotle (1987) *The Poetics of Aristotle*, translation and commentary by S. Halliwell, London: Duckworth.

Barthes, R. (1979) 'Barthes on Theatre', translated and introduced by P.W. Mathers, *Theatre Quarterly*, vol. 9, no. 33, pp. 26–29.

Bennett, S. (1997) *Theatre and Audiences*, London: Routledge.

Bion, W. R. (1984a) *Learning from Experience*, London: Karnac.

Bion, W. R. (1984b) *Second Thoughts*, London: Karnac.

Brecht, B. (1926) 'Conversation with Bert Brecht', in *Brecht on Theatre: The Development of an Aesthetic*, edited and translated by J. Willett (2001), London: Methuen, pp. 14–17.

Brecht, B. (1930) 'The Modern Theatre Is the Epic Theatre', in *Brecht on Theatre: The Development of an Aesthetic*, edited and translated by J. Willett (2001), London: Methuen, pp. 33–42.

Brecht, B. (1931) 'The Literarization of the Theatre', in *Brecht on Theatre: The Development of an Aesthetic*, edited and translated by J. Willett (2001), London: Methuen, pp. 43–47.

Brecht, B. (1949) 'A Short Organum for the Theatre', in *Brecht on Theatre: The Development of an Aesthetic*, edited and translated by J. Willett (2001), London: Methuen, pp. 179–205.

Brecht, B. (1951) 'Short Description of a New Technique of Acting That Produces a *Verfremdung* Effect', in *Brecht on Theatre*, edited by M. Silberman, S. Giles and T. Kuhn (2015), London: Bloomsbury, pp. 184–188.

Brecht, B. (1952) 'Formal Problems Arising from the Theatre's New Content', in *Brecht on Theatre: The Development of an Aesthetic*, edited and translated by J. Willett (2001), London: Methuen, pp. 226–230.

Brecht, B. (1957a) 'Theatre for Pleasure or Theatre for Instruction', in *Brecht on Theatre*, edited by M. Silberman, S. Giles and T. Kuhn (2015), London: Bloomsbury, pp. 109–117.

Brecht, B. (1957b) '*Verfremdung* Effects in Chinese Acting', in *Brecht on Theatre*, edited by M. Silberman, S. Giles and T. Kuhn (2015), London: Bloomsbury, pp. 151–158.

Brecht, B. (1957c) 'Conversation about being Forced into Empathy', in *Brecht on Theatre: The Development of an Aesthetic*, edited and translated by J. Willett (2001), London: Methuen, pp. 270–271.

Brecht, B. (1964) 'Appendices to the Short Organum', in *Brecht on Theatre*, edited by M. Silberman, S. Giles and T. Kuhn (2015), London: Bloomsbury, pp. 255–262.

Butcher, S. H. (1951) *Aristotle's Theory of Poetry and Fine Art*, New York: Dover Publications.

Diderot, D. (1883) *The Paradox of Acting*, translation and annotations by Walter Herries Pollock, London: Chatto & Windus.

Diderot, D. (1939) *Théâtre: Le Fils naturel, Le Joueur, Le Père de famille, De la poésie dramatique*, éditeur J. Assézat, Paris: Libraire Garnier Frères.

Eco, U. (1977) 'Semiotics of Theatrical Performance', *The Drama Review: TDR*, vol. 21, no. 1, pp. 107–117.

Elam, K. (1980) *The Semiotics of Theatre and Drama*, London: Methuen.

Fischer-Lichte, E. (2008) *The Transformative Power of Performance: A New Aesthetics*, London: Routledge.

Fo, D. (1977) *Dario Fo parla di Dario Fo*, intervista e saggio introduttivo di E. Artese, Cosenza: Lerici.

Freud, S. (1908) 'Creative Writers and Day-Dreaming', *The Standard Edition of the Complete Psychological Works of Sigmund Freud, Volume IX (1906–1908): Jensen's "Gradiva" and Other Works*, pp. 141–154, London: The Hogarth Press.

Freud, S. (1909) 'Notes Upon a Case of Obsessional Neurosis', *The Standard Edition of the Complete Psychological Works of Sigmund Freud, Volume X (1909): Two Case Histories: "Little Hans" and the "Rat Man"*, pp. 151–318, London: The Hogarth Press.

Freud, S. (1912) 'Recommendations to Physicians Practising Psycho-Analysis', *The Standard Edition of the Complete Psychological Works of Sigmund Freud, Volume XII (1911–1913): The Case of Schreber, Papers on Technique and Other Works*, pp. 109–120, London: The Hogarth Press.

Freud, S. (1915) 'Observations on Transference-Love (Further Recommendations on the Technique of Psycho-Analysis III)', *The Standard Edition of the Complete Psychological Works of Sigmund Freud, Volume XII (1911–1913): The Case of Schreber, Papers on Technique and Other Works*, pp. 157–171, London: The Hogarth Press.

Freud, S. (1917) 'Mourning and Melancholia', *The Standard Edition of the Complete Psychological Works of Sigmund Freud, Volume XIV (1914–1916): On the History of the Psycho-Analytic Movement, Papers on Metapsychology and Other Works*, pp. 237–258, London: The Hogarth Press.

Garrick, D. (1744) *An Essay on Acting: In Which Will be Consider'd the Mimical Behaviour of a Certain Fashionable Faulty Actor, . . . To Which Will be Added, a Short Criticism on His Acting Macbeth*, London: Bickerton.

Harris, J. (2014) *Inventing the Spectator: Subjectivity & the Theatrical Experience in Early Modern France*, Oxford: Oxford University Press.

Helbo, A. (1985) 'Approches de la réception. Quelques problèmes', *Versus*, vol. 41, pp. 41–48.

Hill, J. (1755) *The Actor: Or a Treatise on the Art of Playing: A New Work, Written by the Author of the Former, and Adapted to the Present State of the Theatres*, London: R. Griffiths.

Holford-Strevens, L. (2005) 'Polus and His Urn: A Case Study in the Theory of Acting, *c.* 300 B.C. – *c.* A.D. 2000', *International Journal of the Classical Tradition*, vol. 11, no. 4, pp. 499–523.

Horace (1970) 'Ars Poetica or Epistle to the Pisos', in *Satires, Epistles and Ars Poetica*, translated by H. Rushton Fairclough, London: William Heinemann, pp. 442–489.

Johnson, S. (1765) *Preface to Shakespeare*, reprint, Gloucester: Dodo Press.

Klein, M. (1935) 'A Contribution to the Psychogenesis of Manic-Depressive States', in *Love, Guilt and Reparation and Other Works 1921–1945*, London: Vintage, 1998, pp. 262–289.

Klein, M. (1955) 'On Identification', in *Envy and Gratitude and Other Works 1946–1963*, London: Vintage, 1997, pp. 141–175.

Klein, M. (1957) 'Envy and Gratitude', in *Envy and Gratitude and Other Works 1946–1963*, London: Vintage, 1997, pp. 176–235.

Lessing, G. E. (1890) 'Dramatic Notes', in *Selected Prose Works of G.E. Lessing*, translated by E. C. Beasley and H. Zimmern, edited by E. Bell, London: George Bell and Sons, pp. 227–493.

McCarthy, T. J. (1997) *Relationships of Sympathy: The Writer and the Reader in British Romanticism*, Aldershot: Scolar Press.

Mounin, G. (1969) *Introduction à la sémiologie*, Paris: Les Editions de Minuit.
Pavis, P. (1985) 'La réception du texte dramatique et spectaculaire: les processus de fictionnalisation et d'idéologisation', *Versus*, vol. 41, pp. 69–94.
Plato (1988) *Plato: Republic 10*, translation and commentary by S. Halliwell, Warminster: Aris and Phillips.
Quinn, M.L. (1990) 'Celebrity and the Semiotics of Acting', *New Theatre Quarterly*, vol. 6, no. 22, pp. 154–161.
Riccoboni, F. (1750) *L'Art du théâtre. A Madame* ***, Paris: Simon & Giffart.
Rousseau, J.-J. (1759) *Letter from M. Rousseau, of Geneva, to M. d'Alembert, of Paris, Concerning the Effects of Theatrical Entertainments on the Manners of Mankind*, translated from the French, London: Printed for J. Nourse at the Lamb opposite Katherine-Street in the Strand.
Ruffini, F. (1974) 'Semiotica del Teatro: Ricognizione degli Studi', *Biblioteca Teatrale*, vol. 9, pp. 34–81.
Sainte-Albine, M.R. de (1749) *Le Comédien. Ouvrage divisé en deux parties. Nouvelle édition, augmentée et corrigée*, Paris: Desaint & Saillant.
Smith, A. (1976) *The Theory of Moral Sentiments*, Oxford: Oxford University Press.
Symington, J. and Symington, N. (1996) *The Clinical Thinking of Wilfred Bion*, London: Routledge.
Veltruský, J. (1981) 'The Prague School Theory of Theater', *Poetics Today*, vol. 2, no. 3, pp. 225–235.
von Held, P. (2011) *Alienation and Theatricality: Diderot after Brecht*, Oxford: Legenda.
Wilson, A. M. (1972) *Diderot*, New York: Oxford University Press.

Index

For Product Safety Concerns and Information please contact our EU
representative GPSR@taylorandfrancis.com
Taylor & Francis Verlag GmbH, Kaufingerstraße 24, 80331 München, Germany

www.ingramcontent.com/pod-product-compliance
Ingram Content Group UK Ltd.
Pitfield, Milton Keynes, MK11 3LW, UK
UKHW022122190926
475702UK00013B/1595

* 9 7 8 0 3 6 7 7 3 6 6 5 1 *